Advancing Health Equity for All

The Robert Wood Johnson Foundation Culture of Health Series
Series Editor, Alonzo L. Plough

1. Knowledge to Action: Accelerating Progress in Health, Well-Being and Equity
2. Advancing Health and Well-Being: Evidence and Collaboration to Achieve Health Equity
3. Culture of Health in Practice: Innovations in Research, Community Engagement, and Action
4. Well-Being: Expanding the Definition of Progress
5. Community Resilience: Equitable Practices for an Uncertain Future
6. Necessary Conversations: Understanding Racism as a Barrier to Achieving Health Equity
7. Advancing Health Equity for All: On the Front Lines of Justice in New Orleans

Advancing Health Equity for All

On the Front Lines of Justice in New Orleans

Edited by

ALONZO L. PLOUGH
THOMAS A. LAVEIST

OXFORD
UNIVERSITY PRESS

OXFORD
UNIVERSITY PRESS

Oxford University Press is a department of the University of Oxford. It furthers the University's objective of excellence in research, scholarship, and education by publishing worldwide. Oxford is a registered trade mark of Oxford University Press in the UK and in certain other countries.

Published in the United States of America by Oxford University Press
198 Madison Avenue, New York, NY 10016, United States of America.

Library of Congress Cataloging-in-Publication Data
Names: Plough, Alonzo L. editor | LaVeist, Thomas Alexis editor
Title: Advancing health equity for all : on the front lines of justice in New Orleans / edited by Alonzo L. Plough, Thomas A. LaVeist.
Description: New York, NY : Oxford University Press, [2026] |
Series: Culture of health | Includes bibliographical references and index.
Identifiers: LCCN 2025044820 (print) | LCCN 2025044821 (ebook) |
ISBN 9780197809419 paperback | ISBN 9780197809426 epub | ISBN 9780197809440
Subjects: LCSH: Discrimination in medical care—Louisiana—New Orleans |
Minorities—Medical care—Social aspects—Louisiana—New Orleans |
Health services accessibility—Louisiana—New Orleans |
Medically underserved areas—Louisiana—New Orleans |
Social medicine—Louisiana—New Orleans
Classification: LCC RA563.M56 A345 2026 (print) | LCC RA563.M56 (ebook)
LC record available at https://lccn.loc.gov/2025044820
LC ebook record available at https://lccn.loc.gov/2025044821

DOI: 10.1093/9780197809440.001.0001

Printed by Marquis Book Printing, Canada

The manufacturer's authorized representative in the EU for product safety is Oxford University Press España S.A. of Parque Empresarial San Fernando de Henares, Avenida de Castilla, 2 – 28830 Madrid (www.oup.es/en or product.safety@oup.com). OUP España S.A. also acts as importer into Spain of products made by the manufacturer.

MIX
Paper | Supporting responsible forestry
FSC® C103567

CONTENTS

INTRODUCTION

When hundreds of people gathered in New Orleans to attend the Partners for Advancing Health Equity Summit in December 2022, the city was almost two decades past the devastation of Hurricane Katrina. The French Quarter was alive with tourists, and many neighborhoods were thriving. Known worldwide for Mardi Gras celebrations, airy, colorful architecture, sugary beignets, shrimp étouffée, and second-line celebrations, the Crescent City has a well-deserved reputation as a place where visitors are encouraged to "laissez *les bons temps rouler.*"

☐ **Play Audio:** Dr. Michael White's Original Liberty Jazz Band kicking off the 2025 Congo Square Rhythms Festival at the George and Joyce Wein Jazz & Heritage Center in Tremé, which is a section of New Orleans and the oldest Black neighborhood in the United States.[a]

Challenges lie beneath that carefree image. Large swaths of the city never recovered from the Katrina disaster. The health indicators in New Orleans, the surrounding parishes, and the entire state of Louisiana have long been among the worst in the nation. Louisiana is ranked 49th for low birthweight babies, surpassed only by Mississippi, and the state's homicide rate is the country's third highest. Rates of obesity, diabetes, sexually transmitted diseases, and opioid disorders are far above national averages. These averages mask very troubling disparities by race. Average life expectancy in Louisiana is about 73 years for White men, but only about 66 for Black men. White women can expect to live about 78 years, while Black women will have, on average, about 73 years of life.[1] In New Orleans itself, there is an extraordinary 25-year difference in life expectancy across certain zip codes.[2]

[a] Dr. Michael White's Original Liberty Jazz Band kicking off the 2025 Congo Square Rhythms Festival at the George and Joyce Wein Jazz & Heritage Center in Tremé, https://www.youtube.com/watch?v=xjvEDwRO9Ug&list=RDxjvEDwRO9Ug&start_radio=1&t=1787s.

But New Orleans has also always been a place full of vibrant communities, and in recent years, community organizations have played a growing role. Determined not to be seen exclusively as a vibrant place for visitors, nor primarily as a city where residents in many neighborhoods live at the hard edge of fear, violence, and poor health, community activists have become a force to be reckoned with. Residents across the city are engaged in reshaping their home in the wake of Katrina, and insisting that the politicians and the business establishment hear their voices and act on their demands.

Advancing Health for All: On the Front Lines of Equity and Justice, the latest volume in RWJF's Culture of Health series, captures those complex truths. The springboard for this book was the Equity Summit, hosted by Tulane University Celia Scott Weatherhead School of Public Health and Tropical Medicine and sponsored by RWJF. Stories of lived experience and additional research evidence from those who presented at the three-day event further enrich the content. Holding the Summit in that location, at that moment in time, took full advantage of Tulane's deep knowledge of the Gulf Coast while lifting up the role that New Orleans plays as a sentinel for experiencing so many challenges across the country. The region—with its rich culture and resources, its aching poverty and enduring structural racism, and the intensifying immediacy of a changing climate—offers a window into the interwoven risks that lie before the entire nation. Yet its rich culture and resources also offer a measure of hope, exemplified by the vigorous, equity-oriented work unfolding along so many intersecting pathways.

We begin to consider all of that with a look at history. Founded by the French in 1718, the city of New Orleans stands on land originally inhabited by the Chitimacha Tribe. The Chitimacha people engaged in a 12-year war against the French in the early 18th century. As a result, many members were enslaved, killed, and displaced south- and westward. New Orleans was an epicenter of the slave trade prior to the Civil War; one out of every three of its residents was enslaved.[3] The economic engine of the South, it was built on the backs of people who worked the sugar and cotton plantations, drained canals, constructed levees at the service of local government, and rebuilt the city twice after catastrophic fires. Its ports brought in thousands of kidnapped Africans, and its town squares served as centers of human trafficking on a vast scale.[4] The Confederacy reigned supreme in New Orleans for only 15 months until it was captured by Union troops, but the bitter war years and the Reconstruction period that followed left scars that remain to this day.

Fast forward more than 150 years. Until very recently, virtually no markers stood to commemorate the brutality enslaved people endured, nor the immense contributions they made. The region has largely failed to acknowledge its past or to redress it in any way. And the scars of the past remain open—healthcare, housing, transportation, education, employment all remain very inequitably distributed. Investments in New Orleans infrastructure never became equitable, whether they originate in the public sector or the private sector, whether they target healthcare, housing, transportation, or education.

The results are evident in present-day indicators that give testament to George Santayana's famed quote, "those who cannot remember the past are condemned to repeat it." Again, a bit of data helps tell the story. Less than one-fifth of Black New Orleans residents (18%) have a bachelor's degree, compared to almost two-thirds of White residents (65%).[5] One can identify disparities in housing segregation, home-lending practices, income, and homeownership in the city. Policing data are comparably inequitable. Black residents are at least twice as likely to be arrested as White residents, including on drug charges, despite research that shows the two groups use illicit drugs at roughly the same level.

Layered on top of all that are the toxic consequences of both longstanding environmental hazards and more recent manifestations of climate change. An 85-mile strip that ends in New Orleans has been designated Cancer Alley,[6] a side effect of the many petrochemical plants sited there. And 28 hurricanes and tropical cyclones—not only the ferocious Hurricane Katrina, but also Gustav, Ida, Isaac, and Laura, to name a few—made landfall in the first two decades of the 20th century, a far greater frequency than in the past. Each devastated the city with rain, flooding, storm surges, and high winds, doing their greatest harm to the Lower Ninth Ward, St. Bernard Parish, and other neighborhoods that have invariably been starved of resources. In New Orleans, climate change is not a risk of the future, it is very much a reality of the present and a dire warning against complacency.

Yet hopelessness is not in the vocabulary of many New Orleanians. There exists a *pride of place* sparked by the musical and culinary traditions that give the city so much of its charm; the architectural heritage that reflects a multicultural mix of French, Spanish, and Haitian influences; the noble history of the civil rights movement; the pageantry of the Mardi Gras Indians; and the creativity displayed in seemingly endless carnivals and parades. Together, these remind New Orleanians that theirs is a city worth fighting for.

Though New Orleans is unique in many ways, its experience of trauma stands as a cautionary tale for the rest of the nation. The immediate threats to the physical infrastructure of the city, amplified by the structural racism that ensures these threats have an uneven impact, affect everyone. At the same time, and far more hopefully, the broad-based commitment to struggle and change in this city serves as inspiration to activists everywhere. The contributors to this volume engage with these themes as they share experiences, compelling insights, and findings that consider how power and policy can be used either to maintain or to shake up the status quo.

At RWJF, we see community power as essential to dismantling racism. Our grantmaking is increasingly dedicated to nurturing community power. Activists who secure power at the local level are positioned to expose root causes of inequity, producing a counternarrative to conventional frames that can inform new policies. Traditional conceptualizations of health, for example, build on a knowledge system that tends to ask narrow questions and sequester data within a medical model. But there are alternative ways of thinking, as the issue of Black maternal mortality illustrates. While a conventional epidemiological analysis would employ a clinical construct, many Black women conceive the issue instead as one of birth justice. That creates a wholly different pathway to improving outcomes, one that privileges community input and ground-up systems change.

A starting point in any power-building effort is to define community, or more accurately to ask people how they define their own communities: geography, history, ethnicity, religion, and gender identity are potential commonalities that encourage people to stand together. In this volume, we consider many kinds of communities and the relationships within and across them that can seed transformation. Local leadership is key, allowing those most directly affected by inequity to determine their own action agenda, construct the research questions and data-gathering techniques needed to pursue it, and establish indicators and outcomes of success as they seek it. RWJF's commitment is to help communities build the capacity necessary to do that.

Advancing Health for All is organized as follows:

Part I: Rooting Health Equity in Place is both a celebration of New Orleans and a recognition of the perils that could undermine it. RWJF's choice to support the convening at Tulane reflected not only respect for the equity-oriented work of its academic partner, but also an appreciation of the school's passionate connections to its home city. In tandem with the powerful attachment residents feel to this unique place, and especially to its diverse, multicultural neighborhoods, this section lifts up the possibility of progress.

Part II: Community Engagement, Belonging, and Power probes the opportunities that surface when historically disenfranchised groups take the lead on the issues that shape their lives. Once, it was commonplace to describe the value of bringing such parties "to the table." Then language shifted to speak of encouraging them to "set the table." But at RWJF, we are increasingly aware of the need to go even further. We may not seek to totally upend the table but rather to build new, better tables by fostering community-driven interactions that build from a position of strength. This section elevates local engagement, authority, and ownership as mechanisms to establish and pursue homegrown priorities.

Part III: Building the Health Equity Scaffold acknowledges that systems and institutions are inclined to preserve entrenched norms, changing slowly, if at all, and usually under outside pressure. But this section also explores the opportunities to redirect their sizable assets toward more equitable goals. Existing scaffolding can be stripped away, reinforced, or rebuilt. Sometimes, science can be a jumping-off point, as when it reveals that the differences in health outcomes by race are only explained by racism, not by biology. Sometimes, it is public policy or academic norms that can be interrogated, deconstructed, and reimagined to better support health equity.

In 2022, RWJF published *Necessary Conversations: Understanding Racism as a Barrier to Achieving Health Equity,* an earlier volume in its Culture of Health series. That book came out of an extraordinary period that began with the COVID-19 pandemic, continued through the George Floyd murder and the social protest movements it ignited, and revealed immense economic and social inequities that could not be ignored. We wrote then that those events signaled "an inflection point in an American journey towards health and racial equity." *Advancing Health for All: On the Front Lines of Equity and Justice* allows us to see how far we have traveled since then—and how much further we have to go.

PART I

ROOTING HEALTH EQUITY IN PLACE

The opening section of this book puts a spotlight on New Orleans and the power of place as an influence on health equity. As the three chapters in this part illustrate, context matters, whether it is cultural influences, buildings, parks, transportation networks, or the risks posed by the global climate crisis that help to define the "city that care forgot." Here, efforts to champion assets while understanding challenges in this most unique of Southern cities have galvanized community efforts to confront inequities.

Chapter 1, "New Orleans Jazz as Metaphor," highlights the city's musical legacy and describes its link to American democracy, the quest for freedom, and the struggle to build a more just world. Through musical and historical references, the chapter contributors deftly convey the creativity, joy, struggles, possibilities, and inclusivity that are synonymous with jazz, making the music a powerful metaphor for health equity. A Spotlight showcases the conference's "Night Out in Central City" with an insider's look at three distinctive community standard-bearers.

Chapter 2, "The Built Environment and Health: Partnering in New Orleans," reveals that jazz is not the city's only equity touchstone. The complex history and present-day challenges of New Orleans reinforce the idea that place is a formative influence on those who call it home. The chapter's contributors address the impact of the built environment on health and well-being, offer examples of multi-sector partnerships that respond to local needs, and embrace the idea of community power. Through the voices of those invested in New Orleans, this chapter emphasizes everyone's right to help shape where they live, even as the climate crisis grows ever more threatening.

Part I concludes as Chapter 3, "Gulf Coast Citizens Take On the Climate Crisis," dives deeper into New Orleans as a stark example of the climate crisis's influence on health, health equity, and the ability to thrive. The chapter portrays climate change as a threat multiplier while recognizing that decisions made globally have local consequences. Contributors examine the impact of climate injustice and environmental crises on water equity, housing, economic opportunities, and health equity; highlight local efforts to embrace "living" and "thriving" with water; and acknowledge the importance of community engagement by those most impacted, including the Indigenous cultures of New Orleans. *Spotlight: The Goal is to Thrive* explores the complexities and controversies surrounding the concept of "resilience" in response to the climate crisis and explains why conference presenters prefer "thriving" as their goal.

1

New Orleans Jazz as Metaphor

Michael G. White, PhD, Xavier University of Louisiana, jazz clarinetist, Founder of The Original Liberty Jazz Band

It is the convergence of different sounds that meet on the common ground of melody, harmony, and rhythm, weaving together a sonic tapestry of sheer magic. It is all there: a loose, yet definite, lyrical trumpet melody with clarinet and trombone weaving in and out in conversational joy. Underneath, the heartbeat, the rhythm section of banjo, bass, piano, and drums drives the ensemble with a steady pulse and a foundational chord structure. Improvisation, syncopation, cross rhythms, bent tones, growls, shouts, whispers, and moans come together as an expression of life in sound, the human experience in all its passions, joys, sorrows, hopes, and fears—boldly displayed and shared through instruments of rhythm and melody.

That's jazz.

And no city in the world is more associated with those beats and these sounds than New Orleans.

This opening chapter begins with expert reflections on New Orleans's signature musical trademark—jazz—and its profound connection to equity. The rest of the chapter is built around the unique perspective of musician and scholar Michael G. White, who takes a deep dive into the history and inclusivity of jazz. Dr. White first explains why jazz has always been a metaphor for equity, a concept he has championed during his long career as a clarinetist, recording artist, historian, and founder of The Original Liberty Jazz Band. He expertly analyzes famous jazz selections to show why "jazz reflects the democratic ideals on which this country was founded," with online links provided so Dr. White's selections can be heard. The chapter ends as Dr. White poignantly describes the power to thrive that jazz brought to his own life after Hurricane Katrina left him personally and musically devastated.

Michael G. White, *New Orleans Jazz as Metaphor*. In: *Advancing Health Equity for All*. Edited by: Alonzo L. Plough and Thomas A. LaVeist, Oxford University Press. © Robert Wood Johnson Foundation (2026).
DOI: 10.1093/9780197809440.003.0001

A *Spotlight* celebrates an evening of sights, tastes, and sounds in New Orleans's Central City neighborhood that showcase the city's authentic cultural, culinary, and musical heritage.

New Orleans Jazz and Equity

The merits of jazz and its unique reflection of the American democratic experience have been captured by documentary filmmakers like Ken Burns in his *Jazz,* described through personal stories in *Hear Me Talkin' To Ya: The Story of Jazz as Told by the Men who Made It"* by renowned jazz historians Nat Shapiro and Nat Hentoff, and debated within the framework of structural racism by cultural critics and *New York Times* writers Nicole Hannah-Jones and Wesley Morris in *The 1619 Project.*

"What you are hearing in Black music that is so appealing to so many people across all races across time is possibility, struggle. It is strife. It is humor. It is sex. It is confidence. And that's ironic," says Wesley Morris in Hulu's documentary adaptation of *The 1619 Project.*

> That's the sound of a people who have for decades and centuries been denied freedom. And yet what you respond to in Black music is the ultimate expression of a belief in that freedom. The belief that the struggle is worth it. That pain begets joy. And that what you are experiencing is not only contagious but necessary and urgent and irresistible. . . . Black music is American music. Because as Americans, we say we believe in freedom and that's what we tell the world. The power of Black music is that it is the ultimate expression of that belief in American freedom.

This conclusion, with its ironic overtones, is embraced by two leading health equity experts, Thomas A. LaVeist, dean and Weatherhead presidential chair in health equity at Tulane University Celia Scott Weatherhead School of Public Health and Tropical Medicine, and Alonzo J. Plough, RWJF's vice president for research-evaluation-learning and chief science officer.

That jazz began in New Orleans makes perfect sense to Dr. LaVeist, a jazz bassist who once considered a professional career in music but instead chose the academic world of public health. He believes that New Orleans *is* jazz. "Jazz is the auditory version of the place, that's what it is," he says. "It's the most unique place in this country because there are so many heavy influences of different cultures—the British, the French, the Spanish. And of course the Indigenous native population that was there before all of that happened, along with a dominant African influence here, too. So New Orleans is this gumbo, this mixture of all these different cultures coming together in this one city. And jazz had to be developed in an environment where you're bringing together all these cultures, because that's what jazz is."

The structure, form, and rules that exist within jazz's improvisational style are exactly why the music resonates as a metaphor for health equity, says Dr. LaVeist. "To me, jazz is about taking and knowing that the structure and the rules are flexible. If you are creative enough, you can break the rules and still make good music. That kind of innovation is what we need to address a complex problem like health equity."

Health equity, he argues, is not simply a medical issue to be fixed by hiring more physicians.

> It's a social, political, economic, and behavioral issue. You put all of that together, and you get the complexity of society, of life. And it doesn't conform to rules that we set up in disciplines like biology, botany, chemistry, and sociology. We try to organize knowledge that way, but we can't fix big problems by just dealing with one discipline. So you need people who are creative, who can bring knowledge together from different backgrounds. That's what is going to be required to address health equity. . . . That is precisely what jazz is. Taking some rules, figuring out how we can creatively bend those rules but maintain enough form and structure to hold things together cohesively while at the same time allowing for individuality and creativity, and make it all still sound good. That is how you think of jazz as a metaphor to explain health equity.

RWJF's Alonzo L. Plough, a jazz guitarist and recording vocalist whose father's family is originally from New Orleans, says he had "always thought of jazz as inclusive. It was always part of my Black community in Kansas City, something that's Indigenous, American, a Black art form. It's inventive, countercultural, and it's populated by major jazz performers who were also major activists in the Civil Rights movement. To me, that's always been an important part of it."

In funding Tulane's Institute to Advance Public Health Equity, Dr. Plough says that RWJF recognized the city's continuing struggles for equity, particularly around environmental injustices that disproportionately impact Black and Brown people (see Chapter 3). He believes that jazz as a metaphor for democratic ideals is best described as something "inspirational, that we aspire to." In fact, he agreed with Dr. White's summation, that "jazz shows us what *society can be*—and not necessarily what society *is*":

> The jazz form, the creativity, the sharing of the lead across different members and the respect for co-creation is very intrinsic to jazz and often not so intrinsic to society. Jazz is inspiration for creativity, deep collaboration, inventiveness, which are all touchstones for equity.

Michael White: Intertwining Jazz and Equity

New Orleans native Michael G. White discovered jazz as a teenager. That's when he played the clarinet in St. Augustine High School's marching band, learned that he was related to such jazz notables as bassist Papa John Joseph and clarinetist Willie "Kaiser" Joseph, and met the great jazz banjo player, Danny Barker.

Now a world-renowned authority on jazz, a widely acclaimed musician, an endowed chair, and a professor of African American music at Xavier University, Dr. White has lectured extensively on jazz as a metaphor for American life and equity. His lectures often intersperse his extensive jazz knowledge with musical presentations by the Original Liberty Jazz band, which he founded in 1981. In these lectures—particularly one delivered in 2010 at the Imagining America's tenth annual conference and another in 2022, at the Partners for Advancing Health Equity Summit[1]—Dr. White also recounts how Hurricane Katrina destroyed his London Avenue Canal home and his priceless collection of 20th-century antique clarinets, manuscripts, and historic photographs. Dr. White's recovery and his subsequent creative and recording successes offer lessons about surviving and thriving in one of America's most musically diverse but climate-challenged cities, noted Nick Spitzer of *American Routes* public radio. "There is no water line on music," he said. "And there is no water line on the soul."[2]

A Musical Son of NOLA Connects Jazz to Equity

> "Jazz is widely considered to be America's most significant, original, artistic contribution to the world, and it began in New Orleans."—Michael G. White, Xavier, jazz musician

To understand jazz as a metaphor for equity, Dr. White first wants people to recognize the uniqueness of New Orleans's other longstanding cultural traditions—such as Mardi Gras, baby dolls, skeletons, and jazz funerals. He believes that the city's Franco Catholic orientation, relatively isolated location, unusual cultural and culinary history, and perennial obsession with pleasure-seeking of all types make it among the most distinctive urban areas in America. In this soup of visual, taste, and auditory touchstones, he describes how jazz evolved from its humble, local origins to become mainstream dance music and inspire the rebellious youthful spirit of the 1920s Jazz Age. But a deeper look, he argues, reveals New Orleans jazz to be much more than just spirited dance music.

> New Orleans jazz is a metaphor for American life. It is an example of, and an exercise in, the democratic ideals this nation was founded upon."—*Michael G. White, Xavier, jazz musician*

New Orleans and Jazz History

Founded in 1718 and colonized by France, New Orleans was what Dr. White describes as a land of "flooding, hurricanes, extreme heat and humidity, diseases, battles with the original Indigenous settlers, angry reptiles and vicious insects." Yet, says Dr. White, the difficult existence, shorter lifespan, spirited citizenry, and Catholic orientation of the settlers also contributed to their special zest for life. This heritage, he believes, inspired the city's reputation for "excessive celebration through good food, drinking, dancing, vice, gambling, parading, partying and holidays [which] took precedence over less important things like business, punctuality, and progress."

An important part of New Orleans's decidedly celebratory nature has always included music. By the 19th century, the city was among the most musical in America, offering European-based music that ranged from classical to opera to folk, from religious music to military and dance music. Accompanying all of this were the instruments, harmonic structures, and melodic concepts that are crucial to jazz.

Another key element of New Orleans's early musical history, Dr. White said, was its Black population, both enslaved and free. "Free Black Creoles often identified culturally with classical and other European-based music," he says. "Many Creoles had extensive training and became performers, conductors, composers, and music teachers." There was also a longstanding tradition of large, open public performances of authentic African drumming, singing, and dancing. First seen before the Civil War in a place known as Congo Square, set within the city's Tremé neighborhood, the tradition has been recreated in recent decades in the same location, now called Louis Armstrong Park.

African-style music and celebration created a rich legacy of rhythms and movements that influenced many musical styles. Dr. White recounts that after the Civil War, tens of thousands of ex-slaves from rural plantations moved to New Orleans, bringing with them the bent tones, call and response, rhythmic variety, and other African American folk elements in work songs, dance music, spirituals, ragtime, and the blues. "New Orleans had the right combination of African and European-derived music, and constant music-related activities that blended and were necessary for the origins of jazz."

Amid Racial Turbulence, Jazz Symbolizes Social Significance

The social and political climate of the late 19th century is another important and often overlooked factor in the origins of early jazz. This period of racial turbulence for African Americans and worsening racial conditions—including the loss of rights and gains made after the Civil War, the rise of White supremacy groups, the increase in racial violence, and new Jim Crow laws that limited Black safety, freedom, and mobility—was reflected in protests, boycotts, demonstrations, legal actions, and, yes, jazz. Dr. White believes that it is not a coincidence that jazz first appeared in the late 1890s, the same decade that one of the most important race-based court cases in American history was argued (*Plessy v. Ferguson,* which enshrined segregation into law for decades).

According to Dr. White, this is also when an uptown New Orleans cornet player named Charles "Buddy" Bolden and others began to use a freer, looser improvised style in playing popular and dance music. Their new music was revolutionary because it reinterpreted several standard musical laws, says Dr. White. For example, though not called jazz until years later, it was mainly instrumental and improvised, boldly challenging standard musical concepts to produce a sound that was artistically flexible. It was also exciting, hot, personal, free, and danceable, evoking a wide range of universal emotions that made it popular among a large segment of New Orleans.

Contrary to popular myth, jazz was not born in the brothels of the city's notorious red-light district, Storyville. The music was not heard only in bars or alcohol-related nocturnal activities. Rather, Dr. White argues, jazz was all over New Orleans, played day and night across neighborhoods, reaching people of all ages and ethnicities through quintessential New Orleanian activities like dances, picnics, parades, funerals, political rallies, lakefront retreat camps, and sports events. Those activities, and the music that accompanied them, helped to bolster the city's reputation for celebration, entertainment, and good times.

In turn, jazz became a metaphor—a living model of an elusive democratic existence sought by the African American population of New Orleans during a racially turbulent time. Says Dr. White, "It is not coincidental that the musical characteristics, values, and social practices associated with early jazz—including freedom within structure, self-expression, equality, inclusion, upward mobility, and collective creation—paralleled basic aspirations of African Americans throughout the nation at the same time the new musical style originated. . . .

By giving people voice, visibility, and freedom, jazz shows us what society can be."—*Michael G. White, Xavier, jazz musician*

Jazz as Equity, in Words and Beats

Dr. White's lectures on jazz as equity often include musical performances with the Original Liberty Jazz Band or the Dr. Michael White Quartet. His musical examples bring his words to life. Pairing Dr. White's language, which is both paraphrased and quoted directly in the rest of this section, with his interpretive jazz selections illustrates his conviction that "the democratic ideals of this country are reflected in jazz."

Song by Song, Exploring Jazz

Dr. White says that the most distinguishing musical characteristic of New Orleans jazz is *collective improvisation*. The music is played in specific keys and has various defined harmonic structures, but within those structures, each instrument performs its role freely. A six- or seven-member musical group will typically include a cornet (or trumpet), clarinet, trombone, banjo, bass violin (or tuba), a drum set, and perhaps a piano. Early New Orleans jazz ensembles might also be small quartets or 10-piece marching brass bands. "As long as you have that combination of a rhythm section and a front line or horn section, that's jazz," says Dr. White.

He uses the *Strutter's Ball*, a popular jazz song, to demonstrate the inner workings of jazz, its root sources, and its social significance. "First, we have the bass, which provides a driving, rhythmic pulse by playing single notes of the basic chords of the song's harmonic structure. The pulse is usually four beats per measure, sometimes accented. The dark, deep tonal color of the bass rounds out the group sound—like on a home stereo where you find a balance between the high and low sounds of the musical spectrum."

Then there is the banjo. An instrument of African origin that was especially important in early New Orleans jazz, the banjo helps to strengthen the group's steady, driving, rhythmic pulse. "Because it can play several notes simultaneously, it colors and fills out the band's sound by presenting a basic range of notes that pertains to each chord as they change, while underlying the melody," explains Dr. White.

Enter the trumpet, whose role Dr. White compares to that of a preacher or quarterback, the ensemble leader interpreting the song's main theme or melody. "A distinguishing feature of the authentic New Orleans style is several improvised passages or choruses of call-and-response-type musical 'conversations,'" he points out. The trumpet typically plays the call, improvising the melody and creating original melodic phrases while leaving space for the other instruments to respond.

The clarinet, the main reed instrument in New Orleans jazz, completes the sound, providing a higher pitched contrast to the trumpet. "The clarinet's main role is to decorate the melody and enrich the ensemble," either by playing harmony as the trumpet leads, playing rhythmic figures to add to a song's driving pulse, or presenting a response to the trumpet's call, says Dr. White. "The improvised musical conversations between these two horns can be exciting, as the clarinet response can take several forms: mimicking, continuing, questioning, mocking, or cosigning."

☐ **Play Audio**: "Downtown Strutters' Ball," played by the George Lewis Jazz Band.[a]

Hymns and Blues

More than a set repertoire of songs, early jazz was an approach, or vernacular style, which absorbed and reinterpreted various pre-existing forms: ragtime, marches, blues, hymns, waltzes, and other musical styles. According to Dr. White, hymns were often played by standard 10- to 12-member brass bands in Black social club and church parades, and in funerals—later known as "jazz funerals."

"A traditional hymn done in the jazz funeral style is *In the Sweet Bye and Bye*. First it would be played as a slow dirge style, mournful and sad, reflecting the grief and sense of loss at death. This music is played during the slow procession toward the cemetery with the hearse," explains Dr. White.

After the burial or "cutting the body loose," says Dr. White, a lively up-tempo song begins—a joyous parade consisting of dancing family and social club members, friends, and throngs of onlookers. This part of the funeral is a celebration of death—the belief that the deceased has gone on to a better place and is now truly free. Here is "In the Sweet Bye and Bye," first as a dirge, and then up-tempo:

☐ **Play Audio**: "In the Sweet Bye and Bye" (dirge), recording by The Olympia Brass Band.[b]

☐ **Play Audio**: "In the Sweet Bye and Bye" (up-tempo)[c]

Another popular style that influenced and became part of New Orleans jazz was the blues. To show some of the range of tempo and mood, Dr. White highlighted two blues songs: "Canal Street Blues," recorded back in 1923 by King Oliver's Creole Jazz Band, one of the greatest ensembles in jazz history; and "Burgundy Street Blues," a slow blues from the legendary clarinetist George Lewis. "For many," says Dr. White, "this song's ballad-like quality conveys the spirit of what New Orleans is all about."

☐ **Play Audio**: "Canal Street Blues,"[d] composed by Joseph King Oliver.

☐ **Play Audio**: "Burgundy Street Blues,"[e] composed by George Lewis.

[a] "Downtown Strutters' Ball," https://www.youtube.com/watch?v=SYf5RtMgUZ4.

[b] "In the Sweet Bye and Bye" (dirge), https://www.youtube.com/watch?v=w-fiJO5_D5o.

[c] "In the Sweet Bye and Bye" (up-tempo), https://www.youtube.com/watch?v=15Zkg_FZF3k.

[d] "Canal Street Blues," https://www.youtube.com/watch?v=y2wM-d-2QOI.

[e] "Burgundy Street Blues," https://www.youtube.com/watch?v=tKL-RJDPH3w.

Social Significance of New Orleans Jazz

The social significance of early New Orleans jazz becomes apparent in both the performance of a traditional New Orleans jazz band and the most popular type of jazz event—the social club parade.

Jazz first emerged in the post-Reconstruction period as African Americans saw their legal and social status and chances for equality become increasingly limited, Dr. White explains. This new music offered a way to express the collective consciousness that addressed social concerns and aspirations for a democratic society. In an era of second-class citizenship, when Blacks were largely invisible in American society, jazz offered musicians social and psychological uplift and the hope of mobility.

Each musician is encouraged to develop a very personal and individual tone, style, and expression, while the strength of the entire ensemble is exalted at the same time, said Dr. White. Together, the team creates a collectively improvised, unified sound that is as unique and recognizable as that produced by any one individual.

According to Dr. White, it is "neither ironic nor accidental that dozens of African American social and benevolent organizations, which grew in large numbers during and after the Reconstruction period, became the principal sponsors of jazz-related activities throughout much of the 20th century." In addition to a number of services designed for social aid and community uplift, these groups frequently sponsored parades, picnics, dances, and other celebratory activities.

Social Club Parades and the Second Line

One example is the social club parade, scheduled annually by each club on a Sunday afternoon between spring and fall. Physically, culturally, and psychologically far removed from the better-known and highly publicized Mardi Gras parades, these events celebrate anniversaries or holidays, mainly in African American neighborhoods.

The traditional social club parade has three components, Dr. White says. First, the social club members, divided into several divisions by age or gender, walk and dance along the parade route. Club members are uniformly adorned in elaborate, bold-colored outfits, complete with corresponding hats, sashes, umbrellas, fans, and baskets.

The second component is traditionally one or more brass bands, with musicians dressed in conventional band uniforms or black suits with white caps. The brass bands play New Orleans-style jazz versions of marches, hymns, blues, jazz standards, and old pop songs at medium to fast tempos. The unique syncopated bass drum and tuba rhythms, and the thick texture of the 10- to 12-piece improvising ensemble, often create a spiritual, almost hypnotic sound.

The third component is the *second line,* a uniquely joyful and completely recognizable New Orleans jazz tradition. "No real New Orleans social club parade would be complete without second liners," says Dr. White. In a second line, hundreds and sometimes thousands of individuals join the parade—following alongside, dancing and cheering along the way. Some intentionally join the second line, some encounter it by accident, and others are helplessly drawn from their homes by the sound of the hot brass band music that can be heard blocks away.

The second line dancing derives from the free-form style of endless movements that originated in West Africa and parallels the individual creativity and variety of brass band jazz. Notes Dr. White, "At times it seems as if the spontaneous movements of the dancers are, in reality, the band's hot phrases and rhythms that were set free and put to motion—joyously leaping from the depths of the instruments like genies escaping from centuries spent in closed bottles. The reverse is also true, as the music can reflect a plethora of sounds that seem like dancing phrases."

To those like Dr. White who know it best, the collective creation and growing intensity of a second line parade takes on a spiritual dimension that challenges traditional concepts of existence. In this euphoric democratic world, Dr. White notes, freedom, equality, and acceptance are threaded completely into the music, dance, and totality of the procession. Age, education, manner of dress, social status, money, physical and mental disabilities, and attractiveness no longer seem to matter, replaced by mutual acceptance, respect, and praise.

One almost surreal aspect of the New Orleans Black social club parades is the transformation and incorporation of objects into "dance partners." Second liners, says Dr. White, are often seen dancing on top of, on the side of, around, and through things that, in the real world,

> might be signs of progress, success, restrictions, or limitations (cars, houses, streets, fences, red lights, porches' steps, bridges, stop signs, etc.). Even nature (trees, wind, mud, etc.), which could deter or halt processions or alter their route in most places, is transformed into a harmless participant in the dance. For example, a hard downpour doesn't end the parade, but merely provides new opportunities to create individual improvised dance movements using wet clothes and water drenched streets. . . . Overall, the second line makes strong statements about concepts such as transformation, power, conquest, possibility, spirituality, overcoming, and liberty.

☐ **Play Audio**: "The New Second Line," recording by The Olympia Brass Band.[f]

A Model for Democracy Extended

For Dr. White, the metaphor of New Orleans jazz and the second line as a model of democracy can be understood by looking at the European-derived march—one of the most structured and difficult forms commonly played in early jazz, which strictly followed a score. The typical New Orleans approach—using improvisation, individual interpretation, collective creation, Black vocal effects, and danceable rhythms—did not completely alter or destroy the strict march form. This powerful analogy suggested that laws in society, too, could be altered, allowing for equality, diversity, and inclusion.

One example of a traditional march that goes back to the early days of jazz is "Panama." The song was written in 1911 by New York-based composer William H. Tyers, and became a popular band song throughout America, played according to written arrangements. In New Orleans, it became an improvised favorite of many jazz and brass bands. Here is "Panama":

☐ **Play Audio**: "Panama," composed by William H. Tyers,[g] played by George Lewis.

Jazz as Healer: A Personal Reflection

Dr. White is the first to admit that jazz offered him life-changing benefits throughout his childhood and early adult years: "a connection to ancestral heritage, individual development, endless challenges, and an open door to the world."

But post-Hurricane Katrina—after losing his home, family members, friends, and a priceless jazz archival collection—Dr. White also realized that this musical life would also help him survive these seemingly insurmountable losses. Jazz, he said, "has helped me to cope in a period of continuing recovery-related difficulties. It has brought a renewed faith, strength, and wisdom that nurtures the soul and brings comfort through a release of emotions and union with others."

Dr. White was one of a number of local musicians and artists offered a "restoration residency" at the artist retreat facility called A Studio in the Woods, now managed by Tulane's ByWater Institute. These special grants were designed

[f] "The New Second Line," https://www.youtube.com/watch?v=oP044Y1K3cA.

[g] "Panama," composed by William H. Tyers, https://www.youtube.com/watch?v=rHraPyW71FU.

both to help displaced artists return home and to provide time, space, and encouragement for creative output.

The residency in December 2007 gave Dr. White a badly needed respite from long commutes between New Orleans and Houston, where he had migrated. Dr. White knows the profound experiences of loss and post-Katrina stress will forever remain with him.

"At first I felt devoid of any creative ideas [but] by the end of this month-long residency I had written nearly three dozen songs," he recalls. "The residency was therapeutic and provided an outlet to express in music my feelings, and those of many New Orleanians, about our evacuation experiences, losses, concerns, memories, sufferings, frustrations, hope, undying spirit, and love for our city."

After the residency, Dr. White progressed from fearing that he might not have much music left in him to producing what he considers his most meaningful recording, *Blue Crescent* (Basin Street Records, 2008). The CD contains a dozen original songs written during his retreat, which explore a new approach to traditional New Orleans jazz using personal experiences and historical events, blended with other ethnic folk music.

> To my surprise, the overall mood of the recording is optimistic and upbeat, and seems to convey joy in positive transition. The other musicians relished and excelled in these new musical canvases for expressing the common emotions that we all shared. . . . Since the hurricane, a renewed sense of the importance of New Orleans's unique traditions like our jazz heritage has taken root. Maintaining and preserving this cultural heritage has become a serious topic among citizens and public officials.

From Dr. White's *Blue Crescent,* here is an original composition called *Sunday Morning.* A traditional style, up-tempo hymn, it is Dr. White's musical message to the people of New Orleans on how faith, unity, and tradition can bring them through the aftermath of the Katrina crisis.

☐ **Play Audio**: "Sunday Morning,"[h] Dr. Michael G. White, *Blue Crescent* Basin Street.

A Final Word

What can one conclude about equity from traditional New Orleans jazz? As Dr. White reminds us, jazz reflects the values associated with freedom, democracy,

[h] "Sunday Morning," https://www.youtube.com/watch?v=sEFYlFPgCQ8.

cultural diversity, and equity, and offers a philosophical framework for implementing them. Just as the jazz funeral reveals the possibility of recovering from tragedy through the process of mourning and offers an optimistic view of loss and transition, so, too, does the struggle against injustice remind us of the power of hope and determination.

New Orleans jazz is at once a reflection of universal passions and emotions, and a local expression of the human experience, said Dr. White. This musical heritage has played a role in the city's continuing struggle for recovery after flooding, racial injustices, a legacy of environmental racism, devastating storms, and health inequities. Dr. White notes that many New Orleanians actually learned or relearned the "value of our unique cultural traditions while displaced and living in places where the cultural heritage was not as rich. A common fear of forever losing jazz, brass bands, social aid and pleasure clubs, jazz funerals, and other local customs is a reminder of a common bond that unites us all."

It seems only fitting to close this first chapter with a song and a phrase used by Dr. White at the end of jazz performances. As Dr. White always concludes, "Won't you join me, and dance along?"

☐ **Play Audio**: "Give it up/Gypsy Second Line,"[i] Dr. Michael White, Live at Little Gem Saloon.

[i] "Give it up/Gypsy Second Line," https://www.youtube.com/watch?v=ENvqMux_EyU.

Spotlight

An Evening of Authentic New Orleans Culture

A recent newspaper article beckoned Mardi Gras visitors to listen to the city's signature jazz and blues along Bourbon Street, dine on braised pork belly and grilled peaches at "N7" in the rapidly gentrifying but historically working-class neighborhood of Bywater, then stop in for brass band night at Bullet's Sport Bar in the Seventh Ward.[1]

A great night, to be sure, but a bit predictable, which is what Thomas A. LaVeist wanted to avoid at the opening of the Partners for Advancing Health Equity Summit. Instead, the Tulane hosts coordinated a more unique New Orleans experience a bus ride away from the French Quarter in the far less visited neighborhood of Central City. Dominated by businesses and homes owned by Black residents in the 1960s, the area hosted Civil Rights activists but then slumped into despair in the 1980s and 1990s. After being spared major flooding during recent storms, the area is now witnessing a renaissance.

During this Central City evening, Summit attendees learned about the city's culinary history with a first stop at the Southern Food and Beverage Museum at 1504 Oretha Castle Haley Boulevard, a street named for the civil rights pioneer dedicated to social justice. While sipping cocktails and nibbling on crudités, the group perused culinary exhibits as colorful as Mardi Gras beads, and featuring kitchen displays, cookbook collections, vintage restaurant signage, and framed civil rights documents. A stroll into the Museum of the American Cocktail, something of a museum within a museum, provided a look into New Orleans's special relationship with ice, its history of mixed cocktails, the world's largest collection of absinthe artifacts, and the recipe for the Original New Orleans Cocktail from 1803 (1 piece of loaf sugar, Stoughton's bitters, water, 2 ounces of either brandy or whisky).

As befits a conference dedicated to exploring equity, guests also enjoyed dinner prepared by members of a youth empowerment program called Liberty's Kitchen. Founded more than a decade ago, Liberty's Kitchen started as a place where young adults who had been neglected, involved with the carceral system, or facing adversity linked to structural and racial inequity could come for a hot meal. Since its launch, Liberty's Kitchen has expanded to provide mentoring, training, and job opportunities in catering services, businesses, and local restaurants to over 1000 youth. On this evening, these aspiring chefs prepared and served shrimp and grits, smothered okra and tomato, Creole jambalaya, and Ooey Gooey King Cake that immersed participants in place-based culture and spotlighted the ways in which food and music can strengthen a community.

After dinner, the visitors and their hosts walked down the street to the New Orleans Jazz Market, a boxy, glass-encased facility at the corner of Oretha Castle Haley and Martin Luther King Jr. Boulevards, the only musical landmark in the city designed specifically for jazz. With an auditorium filled with 370 pomegranate-red seats, the Jazz Market survived an embezzlement scandal in 2017 and, like many once-struggling New Orleans institutions and neighborhoods, emerged to thrive, here as a jazz community center and home to the Grammy-award-winning New Orleans Jazz Orchestra.[2] By evening's end, the musicians, described by one attendee as "funny, exhilarating, entertaining, and musically bold all at once," were on their feet, playing and performing the city's famous Second Line while weaving through the applause and delight of the standing-ovation audience.

The evening reflected the distinctive sights, sounds, and tastes that the Tulane hosts sought to provide throughout the three-day conference, with local culinary specialties and jazz ensembles available at every turn.

> All of this was done intentionally. I didn't want to bring people to New Orleans and have the same conference they could have had in any other city, and typically they only visit the French Quarter. I wanted to show our audience about the city and for them to see the things that are being done to address the inequities in the city, to make "place" and equity as much a part of the conference as possible."—Dr. LaVeist, Tulane University and Jazz Market Board member

2

The Built Environment and Health

Partnering in New Orleans

Julia Kumari Drapkin, MS, CEO and Founder, ISeeChange

Dasjon Jordan, MS, Executive Director, Broad Community Connections

Derek Kauneckis, PhD, Senior Science Advisor, ISeeChange

Emilie Taylor Welty, AIA, MArch, Professor of Practice and Director of Architecture, Tulane University School of Architecture, and Assistant Director, Design/Build, The Albert and Tina Small Center for Collaborative Design

Katherine Theall, PhD, Professor, Tulane University Celia Scott Weatherhead School of Public Health and Tropical Medicine

Ann Yoachim, MPH, Director, The Albert and Tina Small Center for Collaborative Design, and Professor of Practice, Tulane University School of Architecture

Jazz is not the only defining characteristic of New Orleans, where the concept of place has such special resonance. Well-known for its iconic music, spicy cuisine, vibrant nightlife, nonstop celebrations, complex history, and humid Gulf weather, the idea of the city conjures up a dynamic image, even among those who have never been there. New Orleans is a raw, tangible experience, indeed a state of mind, and it matters deeply to those who call it home.

But beneath the pleasures that so many tourists and residents enjoy lies a long history that has scarred Black neighborhoods across the city. A pattern of redlining has left its mark, spawning substandard housing and limiting the ability to build generational wealth through home ownership. These disinvested communities lack the caliber of schools, supermarkets, healthcare facilities, recreational options, and other amenities that contribute to health and well-being.

Julia Kumari Drapkin et al., *The Built Environment and Health*. In: *Advancing Health Equity for All*. Edited by: Alonzo L. Plough and Thomas A. LaVeist, Oxford University Press. © Robert Wood Johnson Foundation (2026). DOI: 10.1093/9780197809440.003.0002

The destructive force of Hurricane Katrina was a pivot point for New Orleans, sparking vigorous reinvestment and redevelopment. It also ignited gentrification in many historical neighborhoods as affluent people without previous ties to New Orleans flocked in, threatening its ingrained identity.[1]

Recognizing the transformations occurring in the post-Katrina built environment, numerous multi-sector partnerships have formed to ensure a community voice is heard in the decisions reshaping the city. These partners share the belief that living, working, and recreational spaces—the homes and offices, infrastructure, parks, and other human-made features—need to respond to local needs. Their work also recognizes the foundational role of community power to further health, racial, and social equity in New Orleans and continue the city's recovery (see Chapter 5).

In this chapter, Katherine Theall of Tulane University Celia Scott Weatherhead School of Public Health and Tropical Medicine opens by providing details about a program that brings together academic researchers, community organizations, and city government to clean up vacant lots and abandoned houses, with the goal of reducing community violence. Next, Emilie Taylor Welty and Ann Yoachim from Tulane's School of Architecture elevate the importance of providing design services to communities that cannot afford them. They explain their design/build teaching approach, intended to develop future architects and designers who are attuned to the complexities of supporting community-driven efforts.

Dasjon Jordan then describes Broad Community Connections, his passion project that is strengthening an important business corridor and improving health outcomes by putting local voices at the center of community-led real estate development. Finally, Julia Kumari Drapkin and Derek Kauneckis describe ISeeChange, a data collection platform that enables residents to provide personalized information on the impact of climate change in their communities.

The Healthy Neighborhoods Project

Katherine Theall, a social epidemiologist and professor at Tulane University Celia Scott Weatherhead School of Public Health and Tropical Medicine, was not surprised by a 2020 report that identified improvements to the physical environment as a key strategy for reducing community violence without policing.[2] Attention to place and design offers a wonderful opportunity to advance health, and health equity in particular, by changing places that have been disinvested in."”—Katherine Theall, Tulane University Celia Scott Weatherhead School of Public Health and Tropical Medicine

As principal investigator of the Healthy Neighborhoods Project,[3] Dr. Theall is studying the impact of upgrading the built environment by transforming vacant and abandoned lots and homes. The project, which is being assessed with a randomized controlled trial, seeks to reduce violence in New Orleans neighborhoods and is based on a similar intervention in Philadelphia that showed dramatic results.[4] In that city, participants living near vacant lots that were cleaned and restored reported significant reductions in perceptions of crime (37%), vandalism (39%), and concerns about outdoor safety (58%). Investigators also found significant decreases in overall crime (13%), gun violence (29%), and burglaries (22%) in poor neighborhoods where vacant lots were restored. Comparable projects in Camden, New Jersey, Flint, Michigan, and Youngstown, Ohio, have yielded similarly promising results.

Also known as the "cleaning-and-greening intervention," the Healthy Neighborhoods Project involves multiple partners. Along with Tulane University's public health and architecture schools, collaborators include the Mary Amelia Center for Women's Health Equity Research at Tulane; the Institute of Women & Ethnic Studies,[5] a national research, training, and advocacy organization headquartered in New Orleans that seeks to improve the health of women, families, and communities of color; Columbia University, which was the lead investigator institution for the Philadelphia study; and both the city's Division of Code Enforcement and its Health Department.

The initiative covers 194 geographic clusters across 23 neighborhoods in New Orleans, mostly in predominantly Black, previously redlined areas that experience high rates of violence and poverty. Eighty of the clusters targeted only lots, 19 targeted both buildings and lots, and 95 clusters were used as controls. Working with the city Division of Code Enforcement, the researchers were able to identify vacant properties that could legally be restored and notified their owners about the project; no one declined to participate. The Center for Employment Opportunities (CEO Works), which serves recently incarcerated people, served as the primary paid contractor for the work. In the vacant lots, the CEO Works team removed debris and cleaned up, mowed the grass, and installed a small fence to prevent dumping. The abandoned houses were cleaned, painted, and repaired on the outside to make them appear lived in, although they were not actually restored to a habitable condition. As of the summer of 2023, the restored clusters continued to be maintained, and cleanup had begun in the control clusters as well.

A National Institutes of Health grant that runs from August 2018 to August 2024 provides most of the funding for the Healthy Neighborhoods Project. The main outcomes of interest under the grant are the impacts on youth and family violence. Primary data come from surveys, focus groups, and interviews with people living in the study clusters. Secondary data provide information on numbers of youth homicides, youth assaults, and domestic violence calls, as well as on child maltreatment.

Additional funding came from a four-year grant (through December 2022) from RWJF's Evidence for Action program,[6] which supports research to evaluate antiracist interventions designed to improve health, well-being, and equity. Under the RWJF grant, the investigators assessed sense of safety, sense of community, collective efficacy, health interconnectedness, civic engagement, and other outcomes that could suggest an association between improving vacant and abandoned property and reducing violence.

To build support, the team communicates regularly with the Mayor's Neighborhood Engagement Office and with community development organizations, faith-based leaders, and neighborhood associations to build support. "Community reaction has been great," says Dr. Theall, noting that researchers share data with residents and provide them with additional resources related to food insecurity, mental health, violence, and other issues of concern. Although partnering with a large number of neighborhoods has proven challenging, local residents have expressed pleasure about the transformation and the role of the city as a willing partner.

Early Findings and Lessons Learned

Preliminary results in early 2023 are positive, including an increase in collective efficacy and a sense of safety. "What surprised us was that residents spoke about the environment and place as being a big contributor to health and wellbeing," says Dr. Theall. "We talk about that in public health, but it was good to hear that coming from residents themselves."

Also striking were the ideas residents offered for repurposing the vacant lots. Some suggestions were conventional, though certainly worthy, such as providing green space and improving infrastructure. A number of more novel ideas were also put forward, such as bringing in goats to graze on the lots. As of spring 2023, the team continues to collect secondary data and maintain the restored lots. They have also begun to clean the control lots, although these will not be evaluated as part of the research study.

Researchers in a number of other cities have reached out to the New Orleans investigators for advice, and Dr. Theall offers some lessons for successfully developing community-based projects tied to academic settings:

- **Take the time needed to develop relationships among partners**. Building relationships is time-consuming and the necessary investments should be made upfront. That way, the trust needed to take advantage of new grant or project opportunities as they arise has already been established.
- **Recognize how long projects take to accomplish their goals, and how messy the process will be**. Because community partners change and cities

evolve, projects are rarely conducted as initially planned. It is important to be able to pivot as necessary, while maintaining scientific rigor.

- **Ensure that researchers receive academic rewards for engaging in community projects.** Coming to the table to shape research in a community setting pulls academics away from applying for grants, writing scholarly papers, and other activities that tend to be valued more in university settings.
- **Disseminate work beyond the scientific community.** Most universities want to increase their engagement with the communities in which they are located, and many faculty are already working on the ground. There are win-win opportunities to share findings and ideas beyond academic settings to reach local communities, city officials, and the public at large.

Continuing the Work

The biggest concern for the Healthy Neighborhoods Project is what will happen when grant funding ends. One possibility is that the city or local communities might agree to assume responsibility for the cleaning and greening. The interest in public health solutions to address the continuing violence in New Orleans increases the chances of that happening, although it would be viable at the local level only with external funding resources. Meanwhile, a community action advisory board with representatives from across New Orleans is considering what can be done with the lots if the resources to maintain them all are not available. "Morally, that's been our biggest issue," says Dr. Theall, her concern evident.

Researchers are also pursuing additional funding to expand the intervention over multiple years and to disseminate findings widely. In addition to maintaining existing lots and buildings, one goal would be to repurpose several of the lots, based on a community-engagement process, to create a "third spot" for residents,[7] such as a community garden or a space for art.

Designing and Building for Health Equity

Another initiative launched in the wake of Hurricane Katrina is the Tulane City Center, which enables architecture faculty at Tulane to provide technical assistance, educate students through real-world projects, and promote the efforts of community organizations to revitalize New Orleans. In 2016, it was renamed the Albert and Tina Small Center for Collaborative Design to recognize its core donors.

The goal is to promote local input and expertise, pushing back against outsiders trying to direct the rebuilding process. "A lot of groups parachuted into town with big visions for what New Orleans should be or could be, with very little on-the-ground conversation, collaboration, and trust building happening," recalls Emilie Taylor Welty, the Small Center's assistant director of design/build. "The people of New Orleans felt like they were being told what they should be by people who didn't even know us."

After focusing for many years primarily on recovery from Katrina, the center has more recently shifted to overcoming the barriers many nonprofit groups face in their efforts to access design services. Today, says Ms. Welty, the conversation "is much more about how we build an equitable and sustainable community that can exist in this precarious place and address a lot of the social, environmental, and racial inequities so that we can create a better city."

As in any city, the built environment of New Orleans is influenced by its history, its culture, and the natural features grounded in climate, topography, and geography. "The buildings and the materials we use and the approaches we take are very much rooted in what makes sense in this climate and in the cultural and historical context of this setting," Ms. Welty notes.

Ann Yoachim, the Small Center's director, stresses the Black cultural traditions of New Orleans. The past and present-day economic, cultural, and social experience of its Black residents all inform the center's work. "The context and culture of the place where you're doing the work makes a difference," she says. "And our work is shaped by the fact that we're in New Orleans, which is a predominantly Black city."

Creativity is also integral to the New Orleans context, as the opening chapter of this volume so amply demonstrates (see Chapter 1). "Art and culture and creativity are a piece of what shapes New Orleans, and so there's value seen in art and creativity more than might be the case in some other places," explains Ms. Yoachim.

> "Art can be used as a means to inform policy and address questions of equity. Public space, art, and creativity have played a role in the fabric of New Orleans for a long time, and that shapes what we do." —Emilie Taylor Welty, Tulane University School of Architecture

Nurturing Future Architects and Designers Committed to Equity

The concept of design/build in construction projects is that the project designer and building contractor work together under one contract. Applied to pedagogy, it is a method of teaching architecture by having students actually build what they design. In the Small Center's design/build projects, architecture faculty and students connect with nonprofits in New Orleans that need design services but cannot afford to hire architects, weaving together the school's learning objectives with the needs of partners on the ground.

"We bring technical expertise to the table, but we don't want students to go into a meeting thinking they know all the answers," Ms. Welty says. As a critical part of a team that can make collaborative change, their role instead is "listening, building consensus, bringing a bit of humility and a bit of collaborative spirit to a project that doesn't just require one artistic genius . . . It requires a whole community of people working together."

As with the architecture field in general, Tulane architecture students do not reflect the demographic composition of either the country or of New Orleans. Just 3 percent of students graduating from the school's undergraduate architecture programs between 2001 and 2020 were Black, as were just 6 percent of graduate architecture students.[8] For that reason, says Ms. Yoachim, part of the pedagogy "is to embed conversations about equity in the design/build process and in the architectural curriculum and emphasize to students their role in addressing existing inequity. This happens through a process focused on changing the project power dynamics and through teaching content."

Equitable Design from the Ground Up

While that equity focus has been part of the design center's work from the beginning, it has become more foundational to its mission in recent years. "If we're only working for the people that can afford it, we're not addressing that equity issue," insisted Ms. Welty. Public interest design, she explained, acknowledges "that the environments around us affect us in multiple ways, health included, and that people should be part of determining the places they live in."

The Small Center selects design/build projects through a short, user-friendly request-for-proposal process, providing assistance to applicants as needed to reduce barriers to entry. An initial 10-year, $1 million gift from Johnson Controls, Inc. supported two projects each year that fit into one of these categories: visioning (design and plan), design and build, and graphic advocacy (visual representation of ideas). A jury of past project partners, architecture school staff, local leaders, and others ranks the projects. Small Center staff then meets with the top rankers and makes the final selection. The project selection process has continued beyond the 10-year gift, with ongoing refinements to address equity and social justice goals.

Before students are engaged, Small Center staff meet with the selected applicants to explore opportunities to involve other stakeholders in order to foster community cohesion. A partnership agreement lays out the timeline and expectations. "This process is essential to building trust," Ms. Yoachim stressed. "This clarity on expectations and outcomes from the beginning was missing in the early years after Katrina. There were big ideas, but not a lot of tangible output."

Because the design/build teams are rooted in New Orleans and actively engaged with issues of equity, people in the neighborhoods know their work and see that they can actually get things done. The relatively modest scope of the center's projects allows them to show immediate results, establishing a foundation of trust, which in turn supports larger conversations around health, housing, and other longer-term, systemic issues. As Ms. Yoachim explains, "We consider questions like: How can we serve as a connector between organizations working on issues? How can our work support coalition building and collaboration? How can we assist work that's already happening?"

The design process itself matters, stressed Ms. Welty. It is a moment to build the capacity of the partner organization and create stronger connections with potential donors, government groups, and other stakeholders. "That can help with people who may be opposed to a project or have had difficult relationships with an entity," she said. "People can learn about an organization, what it is doing and why, and its value in that neighborhood."

Project Examples

The guiding philosophy of the Small Center's design/build team rests on the belief that "each of us should be empowered to shape the places we live, work, and play, and at the heart of that is equity," Ms. Yoachim says. Four examples of collaboration between Tulane and New Orleans community organizations and residents illustrate what that means:

- Working with school and community groups, Solitary Gardens[9] establishes garden beds that are the same size and footprint of a solitary incarceration cell, with plantings designed by individuals living in isolation in prison. These garden plots then become a road into conversations about prison abolition and the inhumanity of solitary confinement.

  The Small Center team worked with Solitary Gardens to design and build "apothecarts," small bicycle carts that carry teas and balms from the gardens to sell at fairs and festivals in New Orleans, creating another opportunity to talk about the work. There is also a longer-term goal of developing an "apothecafé," a home base for the carts and a place to sell the garden products, with space to sit and talk.
- Sugar Roots Farm[10] connects people, particularly school children, with their food systems, raising awareness about how food is produced, goes to market, and affects people's health. The design/build team worked with Sugar Roots Farm on stormwater management and an outdoor covered classroom and kitchen space where larger conversations can comfortably take place.

- After trying several times to build a skate park, only to have it taken down by authorities, a group of young people submitted a proposal to the Small Center to help them design and deal with the cumbersome logistics of gaining approval for the amenity. By untangling the policy, code, and legal complications involved, the Small Center played a pivotal role in getting Parisite Skate Park[11] up and running. "To have a public park that reflects the wants and desires of our youth is really exciting, because it means more kids are out using their bodies and being healthy kids," said Ms. Welty.
- The Music, Arts and Culture Coalition of New Orleans was confounded by overlapping noise ordinances that made it unclear where and when musicians could perform in outdoor settings. In response, the design/build team produced the Guide to New Orleans Street Performance,[12] a graphic[13] of relevant ordinances in a pocket-sized foldable map so musicians know where and when they can perform without being harassed. Police who patrol the French Quarter carry the map on an iPad so they know the rules as well.

  This project "opened up a discussion in the city about the rules and why they don't make sense and has laid the groundwork for more sane regulations and codes," said Ms. Welty. She cites "the power of a little bit of design to clarify and get people on the same page asking the same questions instead of yelling over each other."

Lessons for Partnering between Academia and Community

New Orleans is exceptional in many ways, but the built environment elsewhere is similarly affected by the legacy of slavery and the long-term, insidious effects of redlining. Ms. Welty and Ms. Yoachim offered lessons learned in New Orleans that can inform partnerships between academia and community advocates in other cities:

- **Take advantage of the structural support of a university.** Being affiliated with a university can provide financial stability, including covering staff salaries and the cost of general operations.
- **Understand that projects are embedded within specific institutional structures and local economic realities.** Timelines will be affected by economic strengths and challenges, and the ebb and flow of shifting priorities. A deep knowledge of place and the humility to accept that making change is a long game are essential to maintain commitment.
- **Recognize that academic and community calendars are often at odds, which can create partnership tensions.** Staff members who work year-round need to be involved so that projects can continue even when school is not in session.

- **Be prepared to address other sources of friction.** Differing power dynamics among academia, community-based organizations, and government agencies can all disrupt cooperation if they are not handled carefully. In particular, faculty and community members may think differently about the importance of structuring projects to align with research norms and the value of publishing findings.
- **Recognize the ignoble legacy of many academic institutions.** Tulane University is a predominantly White institution with a history in predominantly Black New Orleans that ties to slavery, the racism of its namesake benefactor Paul Tulane, and the exclusion of non-White students for much of its existence.[14] Confronting that kind of legacy is essential to building trust with community partners.
- **Carve out time to celebrate.** Often the focus is on work, logistics, and funding, but it is vital that all partners come together to celebrate not just the project but the community ties that are making it happen.

Community-Driven Design in a New Orleans Neighborhood

In the Broad Street neighborhoods of New Orleans, new development demonstrates what community enthusiasm and resources can do to improve community health and build equity.

The History and Culture of Broad Street

Broad Street connects six historic neighborhoods in New Orleans: the Fairgrounds, Faubourg St. John (Bayou St. John), lower mid-city (Tulane/Gravier), mid-city, Tremé/Lafitte, and the Seventh Ward. The area has about 40,000 residents and is 51 percent Black, 38 percent White, and 8 percent Hispanic.

The long corridor intersects with Bayou Road, the oldest road in New Orleans and one of the oldest in the United States.[15] It is the site of "The Old Portage," where Native people moved goods from Lake Pontchartrain to the Mississippi River.[16] Those layers of history and culture contribute to a vibrant, ever-evolving community that Dasjon Jordan, executive director of Broad Community Connections, describes as a place in which "everyday working people are able to live and work and be embedded in culture in a very place-based way."

Curiously, the Broad Street corridor is a place that birthed two small businesses that are now national chains. Ruth's Chris Steakhouse began over 40 years ago when Ruth Fertel, a divorced mother of two, mortgaged her home to buy a local restaurant called Chris Steak House. The renamed steakhouse now operates in more than 150 locations worldwide. And then there is the Whole Food Company, which opened in 1974 as a "mom-and-pop" purveyor committed to selling "good, wholesome" food. When Austin-based Whole Foods Market began to expand, the Whole Food Company became its sixth store, and its first acquisition outside Texas.

Also important in the area are cultural and civic organizations, such as the Zulu Social Aid and Pleasure Club. Many such groups of primarily Black people grew out of "benevolent societies" and established "sou-sous," a practice brought by enslaved people from West Africa. Sou-sous are informal savings clubs that were used to care for widows and orphans, pay for funerals, and meet similar needs at a time when Black people were not even allowed to buy insurance policies. They are part of a larger tradition of collective self-determination in the face of inequity.

This rich history has fostered a current-day enclave of Black, property-owning entrepreneurs, many of them Black women. "Now this place has become a destination thought of as New Orleans's own Black Wall Street," said Mr. Jordan. "The spirit of culture, self-determination, community, and community health are all tied together."

Yet the history of Broad Street also includes years of disinvestment that have created dramatic and continuing inequities between some parts of the community, including a 20-year difference in life expectancy from one side of Broad Street to the other. A determination to mitigate these inequities has fueled the work of Broad Street activists for more than a decade.

Broad Community Connections

In 2008, several years after Hurricane Katrina, Broad Street activists began to fill investment gaps in their community through city, state, and national grants. They hosted markets and events to catalyze development, including new businesses, and co-hosted informational convenings to enhance access to resources for building projects and to foster a spirit of collaboration.

Eventually, the work coalesced into Broad Community Connections (BCC), which envisions a self-determined, flourishing community connected by its people, businesses, and culture. Its mission is to catalyze revitalization along Broad Street, center the values of residents in decision-making, and build community power and wealth, with the ultimate goal of transformational system-level change.

"This is not about a single project, but about building trust and relationships," says Mr. Jordan, describing BCC as more of a conduit than a creator. "The projects become the vehicles to achieve the impact we're trying to have." Its core tenets are built around the integration of place, power, health, and wealth and recognize that "engagement is the process, not a link in the process." As on a bus route, "people get on and off at different points. What's most important is that there is a bus, and that it's consistent, accessible, and reliable."

BCC provides people an opportunity to celebrate while they learn and organizes events that give people a voice—and then listens carefully to what they have to say.

> "It's about being consistent, creating space, offering folks some excitement, and helping them see that whether they have five minutes or five hours to give, their presence means so much,"—Dasjon Jordan, Broad Community Connections.

He acknowledges the tension between "balancing the fierce urgency of now and building and sustaining trust." While needs are pressing, it is important to keep "moving at the speed of trust, because we're not trying to solve only tangible issues. We want to change the relationship between professional and resident, between government and citizen."

The ReFresh Project

In 2010, BCC raised funds to purchase a vacant store for what Mr. Jordan called "the most mission-driven use possible." The result is ReFresh,[17] which broke ground that same year and opened in 2013 as a community health hub with many tenants focused on food and healthy eating. The ReFresh goals, he explained, "are about creating healthy and thriving people and places, and being very clear about how health equity is directly connected to economic mobility." Among the tenants:

- Whole Foods Market anchors the project. The Whole Foods at ReFresh is an "urban format" store with a smaller footprint than is usual for the chain. Committed to affordability and local hiring, it draws a diverse cross-section of shoppers. Two community health workers are stationed onsite to guide customers through the store.
- Liberty's Kitchen[18] provides training, employment, education, and leadership development to young people ages 16 to 24. It also operates dine-in facilities, a catering business, and community food access projects.
- Goldring Center for Culinary Medicine,[19] sponsored by Tulane, is a community kitchen and demonstration site for teaching medical students about food as medicine. It was the first teaching kitchen to operate within a medical school in the United States.

- FirstLine Schools, a charter school network, sponsors a program called Edible Schoolyard Project,[20] which provides hands-on education about food.
- SPROUT NOLA[21] is a nonprofit organization that advocates for healthy food policies and operates a community garden and teaching farm.
- Boys Town Louisiana[22] provides youth and family services and support.
- Crescent City Community Land Trust[23] helps to provide permanent affordable housing for New Orleanians.

A coordinator was hired in 2015 to promote partnerships among ReFresh tenants, develop shared metrics for impact, and center resident voices in decision-making. The ReFresh Collaborative is likewise designed to draw the most affected people into conversations and project planning. Using a collective impact model, the collaborative brings together 40 organizations, agencies, and individuals across sectors to develop a common agenda and measure outcomes. The group focuses on ensuring that ReFresh "is a healthy, thriving place for everyone regardless of race, gender, class, and wealth access," states Mr. Jordan.

Partnering Lessons

A set of key lessons has emerged from the experiences of Broad Community Connections:

- **Be transparent about where power lies**. If the distribution of power is not acknowledged from the outset, people may question their sense of agency and the extent to which the process is truly collaborative.
- **Invest in telling the organization's story**. Nonprofit organizations tend to assume their desire to do good is enough to garner support. Stressing the importance of narrative and narrative change, Mr. Jordan urges organizations, and the philanthropies that fund them, to market themselves more effectively to ensure that their mission is understood.
- **Dedicate concerted, ongoing attention to growing, nurturing, and maintaining a strong sense of trust among the partners**. Echoing the lessons learned from other initiatives described in this chapter, fostering trust is critical to success.
- **See the engagement process as core to the work, not as a byproduct**. Both small and large moments of engagement contribute to a project's overall success.
- **Start with questions, not solutions**. Go in with "what ifs?" Ask "why" after a no. Leaving with more questions than answers can inform and enrich the planning process.

- **Go beyond lecture-style conversations to have meaningful dialogue**. Accept the benefits of silence.
- **When racism, sexism, or classism occurs, even unintentionally, name and correct it**. "If no one steps in, people feel disempowered, and fewer and fewer come to the next meetings," warns Mr. Jordan. "Involvement becomes limited to the people who always talk and plan, instead of inviting and collaborative."
- **Ensure that the experts don't take over**. Technical expertise may be needed in a development project, but it is important to set the right tone about its use from the start. To ensure alignment, experts need to understand the community's values and vision, and what is expected of them.
- **When partnering with the government or large organizations, remind community residents that they have power**. Voting is critical, but people also gain agency when they get to know their neighbors and make decisions together about where their priorities lie and how to move an issue forward.

How Climate Change Influences the Built Environment

New Orleans and the greater Gulf Coast are on the frontlines of climate change, with its transformative effects on the built environment. "We are experiencing these changes at a level that is more frequent and probably more advanced than most other communities in the world," said Julia Kumari Drapkin, CEO and founder of ISeeChange. "Heat events, floods, storms, poor air quality, environmental justice, pollution issues, inequity in access to energy or transit—name the problem, it exists here in very stark ways." (See Chapter 3.)

That makes New Orleans the perfect laboratory for ISeeChange,[24] a for-profit social benefit company that bills itself as "a community engagement and data platform for cities to combat climate change." Launched locally in 2017, ISeeChange is headquartered in New Orleans and now has online users in 118 countries, although most of its direct engagement work is in North America.

At the heart of the ISeeChange tool is the goal of providing an easy, low-cost way for community residents to inform taxpayer-funded investments in climate and health. "We are actively looking for how climate data are used, how they can improve lives, and the value they add to communities making decisions around climate and resilience," says Derek Kauneckis, the company's senior science advisor.

Inspired by the weather journals kept by generations of Western farmers and ranchers, ISeeChange allows communities and individuals to enter data about their own direct experiences with climate change. Building on the fundamental principle that community members are the experts on their own lives and understand best what is happening in their own backyards, ISeeChange sees itself as "the mechanism in which that expertise is highlighted and documented."

The free online platform is a response to traditional infrastructure design, which has tended to push data down from the top. It also offers a way to overcome the resource and time constraints that often prevent the people most impacted by climate and health inequities from engaging in the public debate. "Without their voices, experiences, and data, we're making huge mistakes," says Ms. Drapkin.

> "If we don't access those folks who are most impacted, then we really don't have a full picture—and that is inequitable."—*Julia Kumari Drapkin, IseeChange*

"The uniqueness of ISeeChange is being able to capture experiential data that adds the context missing from other community data," said Dr. Kauneckis. Whether reports involve flooding, heat waves, or air quality, ISeeChange recognizes that the consequences of climate change are experienced individually, depending on a person's health, socioeconomic status, ability to withstand risk, and the condition of their home and neighborhood. "It gives a voice to how people understand the change around them and how it impacts their lives."

The data entered by individuals and communities make it easier for community organizations, local governments, utilities, engineering firms, researchers, and others to track environmental changes and flag critical issues. Bringing together data onto a single platform enables these users to identify patterns and anomalies, track risks over time, and inform current and future responses, providing a foundation for enhanced collaboration.

Infrastructure investments, policy, and regulatory changes, and opportunities for public health improvements can then build on these data. For example, the information collected by ISeeChange led to an additional allocation of $4 million for stormwater infrastructure investments in the St. Bernard Neighborhood Campus, a formerly redlined low-income neighborhood in New Orleans. Similarly, data from ISeeChange helped the city of Miami generate $20 million from the Resilient Florida Program,[25] which helps communities prepare for impacts from sea level rise, strong storms, and flooding, to invest in stormwater protections in low-income neighborhoods. And in an on-the-ground example of community-level impact, an online user in coastal New Jersey collected data from 500 residents that identified a significant flood risk in the face of very moderate rains during very moderate high tides, a risk three times that estimated by the National Oceanic and Atmospheric Administration.

ISeeChange has also been used to track the health impacts of urban heat. Partnering with the New Orleans Health Department and local non-profit housing advocates, ISeeChange installed neighborhood heat sensors to track urban heat islands. They compared the location of the heat islands to the locations of high household temperatures, as documented by low-income residents through stories, photos, and other data. The study demonstrated the fundamental connections between housing conditions and heat safety, and helped housing advocates establish and lower the city's first-ever cooling standard as part of its 2023 Healthy Homes Ordinance. A follow-up indoor heat and health study, supported by the National Institutes of Health, is underway in partnership with Johns Hopkins University.

Residents who provide ISeeChange data are notified about who has requested the data, and why. When data contribute to an infrastructure investment or policy change, ISeeChange ensures that residents know they made a difference, said Ms. Drapkin.[26] "If their data is being asked for by one of our customers, we let them know, and it's always for the purpose of using the data to generate response, improvement, and impact." Data privacy is a priority, and ISeeChange has security protocols in place to safeguard provider information.

The ISeeChange platform represents the next generation of interactive, community-facing data tools, and the company won MIT's AI for the Betterment of Humanity award in 2019. The work continues with a National Science Foundation grant that will allow ISeeChange to develop additional AI tools to help cities, engineers, utilities, and researchers respond more quickly and efficiently to community needs.

Lessons for Collecting Data on Lived Experience

Ms. Drapkin and Dr. Kauneckis offer lessons for collecting and using data from the personal experience of community residents:

- **Listen first, and with humility**. It is not possible to solve problems without first hearing from those who confront them daily.
- **Understand that complex problems need a complex problem-solving process**. Investing in social knowledge infrastructure is an important initial step. Critical to decision-making is having access to different types of information.
- **Acknowledge community residents as the experts on their own lives and backyards**. When community expertise is shared with local government, researchers, and outside experts, it can drive outcomes and decisions.
- **Recognize the value of the data provided by people who experience the daily impacts of climate change and other social issues of concern**. Anyone who provides data that are critical to finding solutions should benefit from their contributions.

A Final Word

The complicated, joyous, and challenged place that is New Orleans offers myriad opportunities to test and learn from strategies to improve health and health equity by paying attention to the built environment.

Researchers, architects and designers, business developers and marketers, and software and database creators all bring unique perspectives, experience, and knowledge to a process in which they are "not the heroes" (in the words of Julia Kumari Drapkin) nor "the one artistic genius with the magic bullet design" (as Emilie Taylor Welty says). Rather, they are vital collaborators in local efforts to improve the health and well-being of their communities.

In New Orleans, as in all places, the best approaches are mindful of history, culture, demographics, and physical environment. The lessons learned here can be applied to many other places: Build trust and relationships, acknowledge and be transparent about power dynamics, understand the connections between the work and the place in which it is happening, recognize the personal and place-based expertise of community members, ensure that outside experts don't take over, invest in marketing and "telling the story," and, certainly in New Orleans but arguably everywhere, be sure to take time to celebrate.

Careful, consistent, and creative attention to the connections between the built environment and health can move the needle on a community's physical and mental health over time. Equally important, it can bolster a community's spirit and put it on a path toward a more equitable future.

3

Gulf Coast Citizens Take on the Climate Crisis

Shannon Antoine-Hardy, DrPH, assistant professor of public health, School of Population & Health Sciences, Dillard University

Margot Brown, ScD, senior vice president, justice and equity, The Environmental Defense Fund

Jessica A. Dandridge, MA, executive director, the Water Collaborative of Greater New Orleans

Jeffery U. Darensbourg, PhD, writer, poet, activist, fellow for the Center of Louisiana Studies, University of Louisiana, member of the Atakapa-Ishak Nation

Adrienne Hollis, PhD, JD, vice-president, environmental justice, climate, community revitalization, National Wildlife Federation

Vernice Miller-Travis, executive vice president, Metropolitan Group

John Sabo, PhD, director, ByWater Institute, Tulane University

Between the distinctive sights, tastes, and sounds that make New Orleans so unique, the City that Care Forgot is also the heartbreaking embodiment of what the climate crisis, environmental injustice, manmade disasters, and structural racism can do. Positioned on a crescent of land along the Mississippi River that borders bodies of water stretching to the Gulf Coast, the city is largely at or below sea level, a bull's-eye target for so much of what climate change unloads. From rising ocean levels to tropical storms, from excessive heat to the failure of manmade levees and the destruction of protective wetlands, New Orleans is at the epicenter of the climate crisis.[1]

Shannon Antoine-Hardy et al., *Gulf Coast Citizens Take on the Climate Crisis*. In: *Advancing Health Equity for All*. Edited by: Alonzo L. Plough and Thomas A. LaVeist, Oxford University Press. © Robert Wood Johnson Foundation (2026). DOI: 10.1093/9780197809440.003.0003

In tandem with its climate vulnerabilities, New Orleans has a long and ignoble history of environmental racism and injustice, the endpoint of an 85-mile stretch of land along the Mississippi River chemical corridor commonly referred to as Cancer Alley, which is home to one-fifth of the nation's petrochemical and chemical production facilities. The rural communities in which they are located are rarely in the public eye—places such as Norco, Convent, LaPlace, Mossville, and New Orleans East, which have long faced racial barriers and economic challenges. Worsened by air, water, and soil heavy with carcinogens, these communities contribute to Louisiana's ranking as among the states with the highest cancer rates, according to the Centers for Disease Control and Prevention.[2] The Deep South Center for Environmental Justice, based in New Orleans, has reported that pollution along Cancer Alley "increases as the population of African Americans increases . . . this narrow corridor absorbs more toxic substances annually than do most states."[3]

While New Orleans is a striking example of how the global climate crisis amplifies inequities, it is also a model of innovative efforts to make a difference. This chapter opens by examining the intersection of structural racism and climate change as a threat multiplier with a disproportionate impact on historically underrepresented and underinvested communities.

Next, the chapter contributors fight back against the city's climate crisis image as the epicenter of "all events negative," choosing to believe that solutions are within reach. While recognizing that established laws and practices perpetuate structural racism and impede environmental justice, they suggest ways to overhaul practices and policies with an eye toward a better future, and perhaps to serve as an example to other parts of the country.

Fittingly, a Spotlight laced with emotional outpourings explores the complexities around the word "resilience," and offers "thriving" as an alternative word to describe the needs of communities that repeatedly face challenges and inequities linked to structural and systemic inequality and climate crises.

Structural Racism, Climate Crisis as Threat Multiplier

The impact of structural racism on housing and economic opportunities lies at the core of the inequities associated with the climate crisis. It helps explain why Black and Brown people in almost every state live with more air and chemical pollution and are exposed to greater environmental health hazards than White people; why historically underrepresented communities face more climate-related health risks than their White counterparts; and why underinvested communities and neighborhoods are far hotter than wealthier ones and typically flood more readily.[4] According to a 2021 environmental justice report by the Environmental Protection Agency:

> As a result of historic and contemporary structural racism and discrimination, people of color are more likely to live in poverty; be exposed to environmental hazards; and have less access to health, economic, and social resources; making them more at risk for negative health impacts due to climate compared to their White counterparts.[5]—EPA Administrator Michael S. Regan

The Legacy of Redlining

In New Orleans, the impact of housing policies that once redlined city neighborhoods lingers, decades after a 1935 Federal Home Loan Bank Board marked maps with different colors in 239 cities to determine where to offer government-insured mortgages. Loans to "red" neighborhoods—largely Black and poor or working class—were deemed hazardous due to their "infiltration of inharmonious racial or nationality groups."[6] Though the explicitly racist language was eventually dropped and redlining was eliminated with the passage of the Fair Housing Act in 1968, the damage was done: a 2018 report from the National Community Reinvestment Coalition found that nearly 75 percent of redlined neighborhoods in the US remain low- to moderate-income areas, and people of color live in nearly 64 percent of those neighborhoods.[7]

"Redlining, residential segregation, and other race-based zoning systems like those practiced in New Orleans and endorsed by the federal government created profound environmental, water equity, and climate crisis discrepancies in neighborhoods around the country," says Vernice Miller-Travis, executive vice president of the Metropolitan Group. "People always say, 'Why don't people go live somewhere else?' Because of residential segregation, we were forced to live in vulnerable places, due to the color of our skin. It's not an accident."

Redlined neighborhoods like St. Bernard Parish and the Lower Ninth Ward are among those that have experienced the worst flooding and other environmental injustices over the years. Such relined communities are "the least valued among us, and they were also earmarked for dump sites, hazardous waste facilities, toxic and polluting industries, and freeways that divided neighbors. This is structural and environmental racism," explains Adrienne Hollis, PhD, JD, of the National Wildlife Federation. "Redlining forced minority communities to live in undesirable areas that lacked public investments like good schools and housing stock, green space, trees and parks, and opportunities for economic growth and the creation of generational wealth."

One example is the Gordon Plaza Community of New Orleans, a housing development built in the late 1970s. Described in marketing materials as "a dream for Black home buyers," it proved instead to be a nightmare. It sits atop a municipal landfill, and residents have complained for 40 years about exposure to toxic waste in their yards, corroding pipes, and high rates of cancer. After years of fighting and a class action lawsuit against the city for relocation funding "without devaluation and discrimination," the 60 families remaining in late 2022 continued to hold out hope that the city would fund their relocation fully and equitably.[8]

According to Dr. Hollis, the residents of Gordon Plaza and those living along Cancer Alley are among the 27 million people today who live within a half a mile of a brownfield site, contaminated by hazardous substances that is in most places abandoned, sometimes cleaned up, sometimes not. Take that out to three miles, and you'll find about 143 million people, which is 44% of the U.S. population living in proximity to these sites. That's 58% of all Black people, 57% of people who are isolated because they speak little or no English, 51% of all Hispanics, 53% of all minorities, and 50% of all people with less than a high school education. . . .

> When you introduce climate change, it makes every condition that I've mentioned exponentially worse. That's a threat multiplier.—Adrienne Hollis, National Wildlife Federation

Most people who live in areas prone to flooding, near toxic waste dumps, and in close proximity to dangerous air and water pollution are already part of marginalized communities.[9] Merely living in such places is risky, and when climate change causes excessive flooding, heat waves, and storms, the threat increases exponentially. Extreme weather events can be immediate causes of injury and death or can have longer-term health consequences associated with the spread of waterborne diseases, contaminated industrial and agricultural waste runoff, damaged housing, and disrupted access to food, water, healthcare, and medication.[10]

When Climate Crisis, Structural Racism, and Health Inequities Merge

In May 2022, RWJF published three brief reports to highlight how climate change multiplies the health inequities rooted in structural racism.[11] These studies are now part of the comprehensive research on climate inequity at Partners for Advancing Health Equity at Tulane University Celia Scott Weatherhead School of Public Health and Tropical Medicine.

"While climate change is taking its toll on the physical and mental health of everyone, the burden isn't even or fair," asserts RWJF. "Some of us feel it sooner and more intensely, depending on where we live or work, our race or ethnicity, age, income, or current health. And regardless of factors like income and jobs, there are some communities who face greater health burdens because of past and ongoing policies and disinvestment. For example, the communities on the frontlines of climate change often don't have the same support and resources from government that other communities have—and they're more likely to be home to people of color."[12]

> The health inequities we see today, which too often are the results of structural and systemic racism, are made even worse by a changing climate.—*RWJF, Health and Climate Solutions Initiative report*

The Lower Ninth Ward of New Orleans is an example of this disparate impact and the damning consequences of the government's uneven response to climate disasters. A community known for its civil rights activism—one that previously had one of the highest rates of homeownership for Black people in the country—the Lower Ninth Ward has become "a world symbol for poverty, neglect, and utter devastation."[13] Inequitable disaster recovery resources have made it impossible for thousands of displaced residents to return to their homes. According to multiple reports, the post-Katrina federal rebuilding program discriminated against claimants in areas such as the Lower Ninth Ward by pegging the formula payout to home value rather than the cost to rebuild. The result was to leave many people well short of the money needed to afford a house.

Recalls Dr. Brown:

> When I returned to New Orleans in March 2006 to defend my dissertation, the Whole Foods up on Magazine Street in Uptown looked exactly the same. Exactly the same just six months after Katrina! Flash forward 15 years later, I'm visiting with my husband and my children, we are driving around the Lower Ninth Ward, and there are houses that are still boarded up, and still spray-painted with FEMA's "X" rescue mark from 2005. So a well-resourced area of the city is up and running and back to normal in months, and a Black neighborhood that was completely flooded when the levees broke is still decimated 15 years later. That is wholly offensive.

Those outcomes are not unique, as these findings from the RWJF briefs suggest:

- **Climate change is warming cities unevenly and deepening health inequities.**
  - Climate change makes urban areas like New Orleans hotter, especially for those who live in communities that lack the infrastructure that can keep people cool. Patterns of disinvestment by government and businesses, the history of redlining, and current-day policies such as exclusionary zoning, have created sharp contrasts in the availability of parks, tree canopy, and other heat-mitigating infrastructure. During the "heat dome" in the Pacific

Northwest at the end of June 2021, temperatures between neighborhoods varied by as much as 25 degrees, depending on what public and private sector investments had been made over time.

- The populations most likely to live in hotter neighborhoods are disproportionately people of color. Compared to non-Hispanic Whites, non-Hispanic Blacks were 52 percent more likely to live in neighborhoods without trees and where over half the ground was covered by concrete and pavement, as were more than 32 percent of non-Hispanic Asians. Hispanics were 21 percent more likely to live in such neighborhoods.
- The impacts of climate crisis on marginalized communities can last years or decades. One year after Hurricane Katrina, 32 percent of New Orleans residents said their life remained "very or somewhat disrupted" by the storm, a figure that soared to 59 percent among Black residents in Orleans Parish.[14]

  Nearly two decades later, public health expert Shannon Antoine-Hardy of Dillard University said many neighborhoods "are still suffering from the remnants of Katrina," especially in the highest-risk neighborhoods of Algiers, Central City, Gentilly, Hollygrove, Lower Ninth Ward, New Orleans East, and Tremé.[15] This suffering continues, she said, despite the fact that "the federal government has provided more than $126 billion–$140 billion including tax relief to the Gulf Coast Region, and Congress has provided more than $20 billion in federal funds through the U.S. Department of Housing and Urban Development's (HUD) Community Development Block Grant program to rebuild damaged housing and other infrastructures." Quite obviously, those funds have not been distributed equitably.

The health harms from climate change and extreme heat are most likely to affect those who already live with social injustices and the repercussions of inequitable policy decisions.[16,17] According to a 2022 poll from RWJF, Harvard University's T.H. Chan School of Public Health, and National Public Radio, three-quarters of people in the United States have experienced an extreme weather event in the past five years, and almost a quarter of them suffer from serious health problems, including asthma, cardiovascular disease, heatstroke, or some type of vector-borne disease. More than half of Native Americans (51%) and about one in three Latino, Asian, and Black adults report health harms, compared to 18 percent of their White counterparts.[18]

- **The droughts and heat associated with climate change foster water inequities and threaten the ability to grow food in rural and urban areas.** Black and Latino households already experience food insecurity at twice the rate or more of non-Hispanic White households. As food costs rise and healthy food options become harder to access, those populations will be hit still harder. Recent studies suggest that half the world's population could be living in areas facing water scarcity as early as 2025,[19] with rural and Indigenous communities at particular risk.

- **Climate change makes the air less healthy, especially in communities most exposed to pollution**. While Black Americans make up 13 percent of the country's population, the air they breathe is 40 percent dirtier and they are twice as likely to be hospitalized or die from health problems associated with air pollution as White people.[20] People of color are more exposed than White people to fine particulate matter from construction, industry, homes, and vehicles. Defined as particles that are PM2.5 microns or smaller, they pose the greatest health risks because they can travel deep into the lungs. As Louisiana's Cancer Alley illustrates, communities marginalized by structural racism are also exposed to significantly more air pollution from power plants and refineries because these are often placed closest to their homes.

Though cities and states throughout the US struggle with climate crisis—flooding, fires, and excessive rainfall in California and Texas; water inequity, tornados, toxic spills and pollution in Mississippi, Michigan, Ohio, and Alaska; and heat surges in the Southwest and urban Northeast cities—focusing on climate crisis and environmental racism in the South is especially urgent, argues Thomas A. LaVeist, dean of Tulane University Celia Scott Weatherhead School of Public Health and Tropical Medicine:

> If we're going to address health equity, we're not going to address it nationally unless we address it in the South, because this is the epicenter for social, economic, political, environmental, and health inequities, both historically and today. This is where the focus needs to be. Thomas A. LaVeist, Tulane University Celia Scott Weatherhead School of Public Health and Tropical Medicine

Changing the Narrative

Understanding the legacies of colonization, enslavement, and exploitation along the Mississippi River is key to understanding the climate crisis today, says Jeffery U. Darensbourg, a fellow for the Center of Louisiana Studies at the University of Louisiana and a member of the Atakapa-Ishak Nation. "From chattel slavery to prison slavery, from plantations to plastic production, it is a continuous thread of destruction for the enrichment of a few," he argues. "These histories have a lasting legacy here, and manifest themselves now in the extractive nature of the local economy, Louisiana's leadership in promoting mass incarceration, and the vast disparities in healthcare and life expectancy between neighborhoods."

But environmental activists and experts in New Orleans also sound notes of optimism, given the important steps being taken today to mitigate the impacts of the climate crisis and structural racism. Community leaders and environmental experts like Jessica Dandridge and John Sabo embrace learning to live with water, not to fear it. Long-term environmentalists like Adrienne Hollis champion "pre-sponses" instead of "re-sponses" to climate crisis, with solutions grounded in creating, saving, and replenishing natural infrastructure. Margot Brown, Vernice Miller-Travis, and Shannon Antoine-Hardy point to the importance of community engagement so that those who are impacted most are at the center of climate solutions. And as they promote programs that inspire and support young climate activists, they all join with Dr. Brown and Dr. Darensbourg to honor and learn from the Indigenous people who survived for generations in the region. The remainder of this chapter highlights their viewpoints to celebrate the possibility of change.

> When people think of New Orleans, they think fun, gumbo, Mardi Gras, and then they think we're all below sea level and don't know how to fix our problems. That absolutely makes my blood boil. We're doing more in Louisiana than any other state in the Gulf South to mitigate flooding and climate crisis.—Jessica A. Dandridge, Water Collaborative

Living With and not Fearing Water

Ms. Dandridge sees the headlines: "How to Save New Orleans From Sinking," "How Humans Sank New Orleans," and "As Louisiana's Coast Disappears, Its Historic Communities Are, Too."[21] But then she reminds herself that New Orleans was founded almost 300 years ago, that it is the nation's fourth-largest port and home to five of the country's 15 largest ports, that it is a critical gateway between the Mississippi River and global oceans, and that Louisiana's interconnected system of deepwater and shallow ports work together to move 97 percent of US tonnage. When asked if New Orleans is going to fail, she scoffs, knowing that the city has been an entry and exit point for the country since before the 1803 Louisiana Purchase. It is a survivor.

But she knows, too, that the city's vulnerabilities are very real and the nation depends on its continued health. "I always tell people: 'We are the canary in the coal mine.' If we fail, the rest of America is not going to do too well. It's imperative that we survive, because we control so much in terms of the economy here."

Born and raised in New Orleans's Seventh Ward, Jessica Dandridge turned 16 the day after Hurricane Katrina hit in 2005. Her family's home was devastated by Category 5 winds and the flooding caused by fatal engineering flaws in the system of levees built by the Army Corps of Engineers. "Katrina was a manmade disaster, not a natural disaster," she always points out.

In 2021, she and her mother were riding out Hurricane Ida together when water started coming into their house. "At first, I thought a pipe had burst, and then I followed the water in the dark with a little candle, and I saw that the roof was leaking, that it actually came off in the middle of the hurricane." The trauma of that kind of experience endures and is widely shared. On her birthday last August, Ms. Dandridge sat with friends in a New Orleans restaurant as a rainstorm hit unexpectedly. "You could hear a pin drop, because everyone was stressed. It rains here and people start to shiver. My life has been shaped by hurricanes, water, and testing the limits of human acceptance of both."

"Water Chose Me"

A graduate of Xavier University, Ms. Dandridge completed graduate school and worked with the Rockefeller Family Fund in New York City before returning to Louisiana to assume various advocacy roles until "water chose me." It's fair to say she has leaned into living with water with everything she's got since 2019, when she became executive director of the Greater New Orleans Water Collaborative, a nonprofit organization focused on ensuring "a lifetime of living, thriving, and loving water for every resident." Her Instagram profile is, appropriately, "Queenofwata."

Part of Ms. Dandridge's work involves seeking water justice and water safety transparency in her hometown, "cracking the code on how to get government to implement procedural and distributional equity into their programming." At the Partners for Advancing Health Equity Summit, Dandridge highlighted the local water concerns, racing through an exhaustive list that left her practically breathless: that the utility infrastructure is outdated, that there is no water oversight agency in Louisiana, that just having access to water is considered sufficient for people living in vulnerable communities, without regard to water quality, that lead levels in water pipes in marginalized areas of New Orleans are three times higher than those in Flint, Michigan, and that local government puts additives in the water throughout the city to keep the lead count artificially low, which Ms. Dandridge is convinced correlates with higher cognitive issues leading to despair, crime, poverty, and cancer rates.

Dandridge and the Water Collaborative push for changes in all of these areas because "if we're not pressuring our water utilities, we're not going to get the best out of them and we're going to continue to suffer," she says.

"Living and Thriving WITH Water"

Ms. Dandridge is working to create a new culture around water where the city is "living and thriving WITH water," rather than fighting against it and fearing it. "Sink it, slow it, reuse it, and move it," she argues. Translated? Throughout New Orleans and the Gulf region, Ms. Dandridge partners with coalitions such as Thrive NOLA and Advancing Cities, which engage businesses, organizations, and the city to grow the green infrastructure economy workforce. Together, they are incorporating more green and natural infrastructure into restoration projects and urban design by protecting and creating urban forests, reconstructed coastal wetlands, street-side rain gardens, and bioswales that absorb and move stormwater.

Ms. Dandridge stresses that green infrastructure is a tool for social, economic, and physical liberation for communities that have historically been on the receiving end of environmental injustice. Green infrastructure, she said, can reduce flooding and heat island effects, bolster air quality, improve quality of life and health outcomes, and reduce crime. It also has economic benefits, with many jobs offering higher starting wages and fewer barriers to entry, making it an appealing career path in communities of color.

Ms. Dandridge envisions redesigned streetscapes to minimize the settlement or subsidence of the city's upper soil layers, helping to stop the sinking of New Orleans. And she champions what she calls "the most expansive river diversion project in the world," which would open the levee system for the Mississippi River and allow river water, sediment, and nutrients to rebuild New Orleans and coastal landscapes. These sediment diversions mimic the natural processes that once allowed the river to build up coastal Louisiana and reconnect the Mississippi River to its wetlands, providing much-needed coastal storm surge protection in the process.[22]

"The city is always sinking. It's sinking because of manmade decisions, because we put up the levee walls that trapped water and prevented the system from rebuilding its groundwater table, and we're a delta and a sponge, right? You leave that sponge out to dry, and it's going to shrivel up," explains Ms. Dandridge. "We have to open up these levee walls and rebuild these coastal systems through sediment diversions and rebuilding our wetlands. We have to learn to live with water again."

Gentilly Resilience District: The First of its Kind

The concept of "living with water" was the basis of a transformative report 10 years ago by the Greater New Orleans' Urban Water Plan (UWP).[23] "Before UWP, it has always been about conquering and controlling water after flooding," says Ms. Dandridge. "Residents and leadership had never been asked to partner *with* the land and prioritize it in planning and development. It has been hugely successful at creating a new culture around land use, development, and climate adaptation. And the UWP put the ideas of green infrastructure and stormwater management in the hands of the community and residents. Unlike most cities, it has not been top down, but rather bottom up."

According to Ms. Dandridge, the Urban Water Plan provided the basis for the Gentilly Resilience District, the first such district in New Orleans, which was funded with more than $141 million in federal funds after Hurricane Isaac in 2012.[24] Community input has been key to the ongoing projects that aim to reduce flooding, slow land subsidence, incorporate stormwater management, and encourage neighborhood revitalization by adopting new approaches to water management:

- **Blue and Green Corridors project between London Avenue Canal and Franklin Avenue in Gentilly**, began construction in the fall of 2023. The project will use the grounds along major boulevards and between streetscapes to create canals that slow and store stormwater while offering safe spaces to travel and play.
- **Dillard Wetlands, a 27-acre, largely undisturbed woodland area on the western side of the London Avenue Canal**, will be retrofitted to capture water from neighboring areas and serve as a nature preserve and park that supports recreation, biodiversity, and ecosystem restoration. Construction is underway and will include public art and water features to enhance public understanding about living with water.
- **Mirabeau Water Garden, a 25-acre former site of the Sisters of Saint Joseph convent**, is designed to store up to 10 million gallons of stormwater while also serving as a space for recreation and environmental learning.
- **Pontilly Neighborhood Stormwater Network—Phase II/Sawyer Canal Public Improvements**. Enhancements to the Dwyer Canal, combined with vacant lots, streets, and alleyways, are designed to capture stormwater and beautify the Pontchartrain Park and Gentilly Woods neighborhoods.

Ms. Dandridge believes that the Gentilly Resiliency District "has successfully created a narrative and concept that all levels of government and community have deep buy-in into. And it helps us learn to say, 'We love water.' Obviously, we can't live without it, but we haven't really learned to love it, because of the negative experiences we've had."

Thriving ByWater, Wetlands Restoration, Community Engagement

The themes espoused by Ms. Dandridge and reflected in projects like the Gentilly Resiliency District—living with water, adaptive reuse, community engagement, respecting history—are reinforced by many other initiatives in the area, including at Tulane University.

Tulane's Thriving ByWater Institute and Partners for Advancing Health Equity

A nationally recognized environmental research institute, Tulane's ByWater Institute and its ongoing work on sustainability and adaptability have taken on new urgency in the face of climate change, sea level rise, and evolving natural and technological hazards, according to director John Sabo, PhD.[25]

"Industrial and agricultural pollution. Equity of access to drinking water and sanitation. Sea level rise and coastal resilience," states Dr. Sabo. "These are among the most pressing water issues facing the United States. It's time to get serious about addressing them—which means finding solutions at scales that matter."

Similar to Ms. Dandridge, Dr. Sabo believes that cities, coastlines, and river basins like those in and around New Orleans must "flex and extend with nature, rather than resisting it" in an era of increasing climate extremes. Using the Mississippi River Basin as its testing ground, ByWater's "thriving by water" approach is focused on designing, sharing, and growing neighborhoods, landscapes, and technologies that revolve around water. It seeks to advance what Dr. Sabo calls "clinical trials for planetary health" at unprecedented speeds and scales, a nod to the world's growing water problems.

Take the fact that New Orleans is sinking. Roughly 50 percent of the city is below sea level, due to a combination of failed engineering and levee systems, rising sea levels, and crucial sediment supplies diverted from the Mississippi River.[26] "One of the reasons we are sinking is how we manage flood water but also groundwater," says Dr. Sabo. "If there is a big storm coming, we pump the groundwater out so there is room in the aquifer to absorb that extra water. But that makes the soil compact, causing the ground to sink. We have to figure out a better way to manage that groundwater, rather than watching the city sink."

The ByWater Institute studies how to create natural infrastructure by rehabilitating forests to provide more protection and absorb more water, and by reconfiguring or rebuilding the aging levee system so that water and river sediment can travel to regenerate coastal land loss. "In designing that natural infrastructure from neighborhood to watershed, we have to think about that distribution through the lens of equity," Dr. Sabo says.

Another example: Noting that various groups are working to make New Orleans and Louisiana a hub for hydrogen energy production—bolstered by government grants and tax credits to lure manufacturers of clean energy and technology products[27]—Dr. Sabo has proposed that ByWater "partner to invent nature-based technologies that connect waste, wastewater, shipping and commerce to create hydrogen as clean fuel." Although the technology won't be available tomorrow, nor even within a few years, a 10-year horizon could be realistic. "There is a lot of promise for that," he says, hopefully.

Though the ByWater Institute's research-driven program is relatively new and still developing, Dr. Sabo also plans to steer research into what he calls "the public health room," a step that he believes will motivate communities to embrace climate action and form collaborations across medicine and climate science. "As climate changes and climate warms, the range of tropical disease is going to march north," he warns, noting that a recently announced National Institutes of Health grant will enhance this research.

> Malaria, dengue fever, those diseases you think of as tropical are going to be more frequently observed in temperate climates that are becoming warmer. . . . Climate and water problems that we are facing today—sea-level rise, dead zones, coastal land loss, and equitable access to environmentally safe spaces—are the cholera and malaria of the 21st century. Planning for greater resilience and adaptability has taken on a sense of urgency in New Orleans and other coastal communities in the face of climate change.—John Sabo, ByWater Institute, Tulane University

In addition to the ByWater Institute, many divisions at Tulane are focused on climate and water issues, including the Tulane Institute on Water Resources Law and Policy and Partners for Advancing Health Equity, where Dr. LaVeist has prioritized climate change research. He is also working to transition the school's Department of Environmental Health Sciences to focus on climate change and its inequitable impact on health as well as on environmental justice. From recruiting new faculty to partnering with other departments in the School of Science & Engineering and the School of Architecture, Dr. LaVeist notes that he is "looking broadly at other disciplines we'll need to collaborate with to fully understand the complexity of these problems."

Is it enough? Is Dr. LaVeist worried about the future of New Orleans? "I'm not terrified, but I do think about it," he admits, adding, with a touch of irony, "I mean, I live in a city that is below sea level and surrounded by water. What could go wrong?"

Dr. Sabo offered his favorite sandwich analogy to explain that while New Orleans is going to survive into the future, it will become a very different place:

> There are people and businesses, the economically disadvantaged, which tend to be Brown and not White, that's the bottom supportive layer, the very foundation of the community, and they aren't leaving. The big companies (i.e., oil and gas industries, medical centers, universities) have their infrastructure here and it would cost them billions to go, so that's the top layer and they aren't leaving. So what's impacted the most is the stuff in the middle, all the services, restaurants, police, power and water services, arts, schools. How do we devote more resources to the city to make sure those critical services are here, such that we can thrive? That's the million-dollar question.

Restoration for Wetlands

Louisiana's coastal habitat is home to one of the nation's largest commercial fisheries and shellfish nurseries, second only to Alaska. It is also the state's first line of defense during storms, reducing the effects of wind, waves, and flooding. But over time, the development of shipping canals and levees, coupled with devastating Gulf Coast oil spills, storms, and rising sea levels, have threatened or destroyed hundreds of thousands of acres of Louisiana wetlands. Unless drastic measures were taken, the National Oceanic and Atmospheric Administration (NOAA) predicted in 2022 that the Louisiana coastline would move inland by 33 miles during the lifetime of a child born that year, erasing approximately 800,000 acres of wetlands.[28]

Some progress has been made to alter that bleak prospect. According to NOAA, over 40 wetland restoration projects have been completed since 1990, restoring more than 12,500 acres of Louisiana coastal habitat.[29] But efforts to protect wetlands remain difficult and sometimes controversial. Coastal restoration projects—such as the $2 billion Mid-Barataria Sediment Diversion Project in an area critically damaged by the 2010 DeepWater Horizon oil spill and considered the cornerstone in the state's 50-year, $50 billion effort to prevent the bottom third of Louisiana from disappearing into the Gulf of Mexico—have consistently stalled.[30]

Here, too, there are signs of change. A $600 million award from the National Fish and Wildlife Foundation in 2023 will support construction of the Mid-Barataria project and help reverse the historic loss of wetlands.[31] "Communities in Louisiana are not giving up. *We* are not giving up," emphasizes the National Wildlife Federation's Adrienne Hollis.

The first of 12 priorities in the federation's "Rebuilding Stronger" plan to protect against extreme storms is to "prioritize natural infrastructure solutions for hazard risk reductions." According to Dr. Hollis, that means creating healthy wetlands, upland forests, floodplains, grasslands, dunes, and other natural systems that buffer communities from storm surges and help retain water to prevent flooding. These steps, she notes, ground solutions in creating, saving, and replenishing natural infrastructure. Typically, they also provide wildlife habitat, cost less than structural measures, and avoid the risk of catastrophic failures of levees, floodwalls, and dams.

Why wetlands? According to the National Wildlife Federation, "a one-acre wetland can store about three-acre feet of water, or one million gallons." For example, wetlands prevented $625 million in flood damages during Superstorm Sandy in the 12 affected coastal states, and reduced damages by 20 to 30 percent in the four states with the greatest wetland coverage. In addition, forested and other wetland vegetation slow the speed of flood waters and, when combined with wetland flood storage, lower flood heights.[32]

On one of her recent visits to Louisiana, Dr. Hollis recalls, "I saw and heard about people working to reclaim wildlife areas, to re-establish natural plants, natural trees that absorb not only the extra water but pollutants, too. It has to be endemic to the area. We have to stop taking a natural area that was created for one thing and using it for something else." At the end of the day, she says, nature will reassert itself and determine what the land will become.

> We are welcoming nature home, that's really what we are doing. – Adrienne Hollis, National Wildlife Federation

Indigenous Knowledge and Sacrifice

Ms. Dandridge is quick to note that the concept of "living with water" is rooted in the area's ancestral and Indigenous roots, going back to the 22 tribes that lived in Louisiana before the French arrived. Dr. Darensbourg also points out that Indigenous people are among the very first environmentalists—respecting both coastal and inland areas, using their resources in ways that protect them, and promoting environmental justice.

But today's wetlands restoration efforts are often too little, too late, for many of Louisiana's coastal Indigenous communities. Brown's poignant story about one such community—the Isle de Jean Charles Biloxi-Chitimacha-Choctaw Tribe, located about 50 miles south of New Orleans along the Gulf—involved what she calls "structural racism, environmental injustice, and climate change."

As Dr. Brown recounts, the federal government displaced and scattered more than 60,000 Indigenous people from northern areas of Arkansas, Mississippi, and Alabama, and regions west of the Mississippi River almost 200 years ago. Recovering from hardship and heartache, some of them were able to rebuild in the Gulf area of Isle de Jean Charles, creating what Brown calls "an incredibly rich culture and thriving community." Now that, too, has been decimated as rising sea levels have claimed 98 percent of their land. With their homes uninhabitable, they've been forced to relocate dozens of miles inland.

> The Isle de Jean Charles Biloxi-Chitimacha-Choctaw Tribe may be the first community that was relocated in Louisiana. I can assure you it will not be the last, –Margot Brown, Environmental Defense Fund.

Similar stories of forced climate migration are becoming more common among Indigenous communities. During Hurricane Ida, the Pointe-au-Chien and Houma tribes were devastated by the destruction of whole neighborhoods of Indigenous people in Terrebonne Parish. In 2020, according to Dr. Darensbourg, Hurricanes Delta and Laura caused many of his own tribal members to lose their homes, too.

What storms and the climate crisis don't destroy along the coastline, oil and shipping companies often do. Consider the significance of the shell midden destruction in the middle of Four Mile Cut, where the Vermilion River empties into the Gulf of Mexico in Vermilion Parish. "A shell midden is what we created there with a range of clamshells, gleaming, white shells from on the shore," explains Dr. Darensbourg. "This is sacred ground to the Atakapa-Ishak Nation of Indians, a marker for where the village would be. Our chiefs are buried here. And now this 600-meters-long structure has a ship channel cutting right through it to allow boats to get out to oil rigs. This sacred, historical marker is cut in twain for the petroleum industry, designed and built to allow boats to get out to oil rigs. And we can do nothing about it."

Ignoring Indigenous knowledge and experience causes long-lasting harm not only to Indigenous peoples and Nations but to the entire population, says Dr. Brown. Pointing to the failed levee system, Dr. Brown argues that "there was extensive Indigenous knowledge in the bayous when those levees were put up, but no one consulted with the communities that had lived there for hundreds of years. They knew how the creeks flowed, they knew how the bayous worked. The lack of understanding, the blatant ignorance on the part of the US government in dismissing their intellectual capacity and historical knowledge has resulted in where we are today in southern Louisiana."

This pattern of dismissing Indigenous wisdom is not new, Dr. Darensbourg explains. He tells a tribal story from 1831 about a hurricane approaching Grand Chenier in Cameron Parish. "A member of my tribe warned a White family living nearby that he had detected an approaching storm by reading signs in the water, and that they should follow us into some trees we had prepared for storms where we would strap ourselves in with vines to survive the surging winds and water. That White family ignored this advice, and they drowned.[33] . . .

> We are still warning people about a coming storm, coming calamity, and still Indigenous people bear witness to different ways of life that can save humanity. Will others listen? The hurricane is approaching. *–Jeffery U. Darensbourg*

Community Engagement

The stories of those fighting back against inequity and injustice help illustrate the importance of community engagement, which is discussed in-depth in Part II of this book. Here, the chapter contributors look briefly at the concept in the context of climate change.

Dillard University's Dr. Shannon Antoine-Hardy believes that climate change needs to be considered not only on a global level, but also on a community or individual level. From a socio-ecological perspective, she argues, "individual characteristics of a local government's resources, political structure, and community attributes will help identify a unique set of needs and opportunities to devise an action plan that will address the impacts of climate change at every level. People need to be involved in the conversation when it comes down to developing environmental policies, regulations, laws that will affect our lives. It needs to be more inclusive."

One way to bring in those voices is through community-based participatory research, where both researchers and community stakeholders—among them, residents, climate and environmental activists, and government representatives—engage as equal partners to create feasible climate action plans. "If one of our goals is to truly rectify these climate-related health and social inequities triggered by structure racism, we need to include the very people who are the recipients of redlining and neighborhood segregation," says Dr. Antoine-Hardy.

Her own research agenda, focused on reducing environmental pollutants and mitigating the impacts of climate change, emphasizes the importance of "understanding the role of policy, systems, and environmental changes strategies and their influence on social determinants of health among marginalized, minority-based populations."

Cancer Alley is prime territory for her work because the siting of petrochemical plants is clearly no coincidence. "Where are those plants located?," she asked. "Not in the prestigious, gated golf course communities; they are located in the low-income neighborhoods primarily occupied by Black and Brown people." In planning for community engagement, that makes it "crucial to examine the historical and economic conditions of each impacted community to evaluate the problem areas such as resource extraction, inheritance pollution, waste and recycling services, and accessibility to sustainable transportation."

Ms. Miller-Travis agrees on the importance of having the kind of conversations emphasized by Dr. Antoine-Hardy, noting the obligation to "bring people into the room who have that lived experience, and believe them. And then figure out a way to wrap that into whatever your analysis is and what your research models are." Dr. Hollis argues for going even further: "Don't just put them in the room—have them lead the conversation."

The value of doing just that became dramatically apparent to Dr. Brown as she worked with the Biloxi-Chitimacha-Choctaw Tribe after they were forced to migrate from the Isle de Jean Charles. Practicing what she called "radical listening" helped her understand that the "people closest to the problem are also the people closest to the solution." It also revealed that her original plan to help the tribe create a healthcare center as a driver for economic revitalization did not align with the community's priorities or needs.

"It was not what they wanted, nor was it what they needed," she says. "What I learned, in talking and listening to these members of the tribe, was the sadness they were experiencing through the loss of culture and their ancestral community. So they coined a construct called 'the Preservation of Place.' Now, they'll be building their own museum, something that best addresses the mental health and wellbeing of the community and helps preserve their culture."

In a place like New Orleans, which has a complicated relationship with the oil industry, people often disagree on who should be heard when the topic is the climate crisis. Ms. Dandridge does not want fossil fuel companies involved, even though she recognizes the huge economic impact they have in the region. Dr. Sabo, a former business consultant, feels differently because he does not see how progress against the climate crisis can be made unless oil and gas representatives have a say. This debate took on greater urgency in early 2023 when the governor of Louisiana announced a fully funded, $1.8 billion project to build a new container terminal on the Lower Mississippi River. Located just below a metal bridge that huge container ships were unable to navigate, it will open the port to much larger transport ships, putting the city back in play with the largest supply chain purveyors.[34] Yet to be determined is the project's potential to undermine efforts to re-establish valuable wetlands.

Dr. Hollis believes simply that "everyone plays a role. We have to have all stakeholders engaged. But the [fossil fuel companies] have to realize and acknowledge what bad decisions they have made, generally focused on profit over people. The only way to change that is to get them involved. In an equitable manner, you need everyone to get to the table."

A Final Word

The challenges ahead cannot be minimized, but the considerable efforts underway to mitigate structural racism and reverse the trajectory of the climate crisis still need to be celebrated. At the federal level, the Biden Administration pursued multiple infrastructure projects, climate crisis initiatives, and executive actions, bringing hope for progress through environmentally sound and sustainable measures. A regional initiative of interest is the partnership between the Gulf Research Program and RWJF, which is designed to advance health equity in at-risk Gulf Coast communities by improving public health data systems in areas that are disproportionately experiencing the impacts of climate change.[35]

Locally, the quality of drinking water will likely be informed in the coming years by the Water Collaborative's report on "forever chemicals" in Cancer Alley, which includes recommendations for community coalition engagement, continued advocacy for legislative initiatives to fight pollution, and methods to personally reduce exposure to harmful chemical in drinking water.[36]

Neighborhood-level activities include efforts by the DeepSouth Center for Environment Justice and the Lower Ninth Ward's Sankofa Community Development Corporation, who are working together to support the development of the Sankofa Wetland Park and Nature Trail. This long-term recovery project is designed to protect the Lower Ninth Ward from hurricanes and flooding while creating a community asset with green infrastructure in an area once known best for blight and illegal dumping. With 32 remaining acres, Sankofa recently partnered with the city to develop the space for outdoor activities like fishing, canoeing, biking, and more.[37]

Such progress is gaining national attention. Instead of the usual headlines focused on flooding in New Orleans, a recent *New York Times* travel article reflected the very "living with water" concepts championed by Ms. Dandridge and Dr. Sabo. With a nod to "new ways to engage with the city's history, arts scene, and natural beauty," the piece highlighted both the environmentally friendly biking and pedestrian path called Lafitte Greenway in City Park and the Bayou St. John's transformation into an ecologically-restored waterway for turtles, egrets, pelicans, and kayak paddlers.[38]

Dr. LaVeist remains realistic but hopeful. And he believes that lessons to finding solutions for climate crisis issues in the region can be taken from that quintessentially New Orleans sound described in the opening chapter—jazz (see Chapter 1). "That kind of innovation, that creativity, is what we need to address a complex problem like climate crisis."

Spotlight

The Goal is to Thrive

In a Partners for Advancing Health Equity Summit discussion, "Climate, Disasters, and the Future of Health in Gulf Cities," Jeffery Darensbourg briefly touched on the concept of resilience in Native tribes such as his own Atakapa-Ishak Nation. "We live by the tenet that you take care of your people, you thrive," he said. "So when we are called upon to be resilient, well, we're already resilient. It would be nice to need to be less resilient so that we can focus on other things for a bit."

Moderator John Sabo then asked if the terms "resilience" and "thriving" are "completely different things? Like 'thriving' is better than just being 'resilient?'"

The tension in the room was palpable.

"Can we cancel the word 'resilience'?" asked panelist Jessica Dandridge. "It has harmed us. It has meant that Brown and Black people, Indigenous and other minority groups are forced to struggle longer and harder with less. That's what that means."

To the sound of applause and an "Amen," Dandridge continued, her typically rapid speech becoming progressively faster: "To say one is resilient, says that, 'oh, you can bear the brunt and the violence and the pain over and over again, but I'm not going to give you what you need to thrive.' We want to be on the other end of that conversation, thriving. Which is when we have enough resources, our community is strong, everybody in our community matters and everyone in our community can participate. Everyone in our community can have healthy living, whether that be the water, the food, the air. Thriving means that I can be one with the land, whether it be our physical land, our urban built environment infrastructure systems. That is where we have to go if we're going to talk about disaster and the future of our cities."

Dandridge wasn't done. "It's no longer about resilience. We've studied that over and over again. We've looked at every report and all the people that we looked at are people who aren't thriving. So is resiliency actually working? When we use that term, is it actually building better cities or is it harming cities? We need to think about sustainability and building equity and equality into our infrastructure systems at a state and city level. And again, really addressing the core of why we as a country struggle with thriving. We have to understand the cause and effect. And I know it's hard for some people when you say the word "colonization" or we talk about White supremacy—they shrink up. But we are here, in 2022, in the political and social environment we have, because we haven't addressed the core underlying problems."

> So I ask the audience, the next time you see the word "resilient," scratch it out on the report and put in "thrive."—Jessica Dandridge, The Water Collaborative

Similar heated conversations were heard throughout the New Orleans conference, especially during a panel discussion on "Climate Change as a Threat Multiplier." Panel moderator Adrienne Hollis agreed that wordsmithing is critical in order to move forward equitably.

"We already know that people are resilient," said Hollis. "We've been resilient since slavery. You don't want people to always be in situations where they have to bounce back—because you can't expect to move forward if you are always recovering. So we want every person to be protected. We have to want to mitigate the problems faced by those who are disproportionately impacted by poverty, climate change, lack of access to healthcare. Instead of looking at an issue and generating a response, a 'pre-sponse' is better. That helps communities thrive—and not just survive."

RWJF's Alonzo L. Plough agreed. "I'm much more about communities thriving and recognizing the natural ability to thrive that they demonstrate every day," he said. "I think that word choice is better."

Though "resilience" remains part of the Foundation's lexicon, and was often said casually at the conference, its use is increasingly being questioned. Dr. Plough said that he personally has stopped using the word, recognizing that it carries a lot of baggage. "We need to be very careful in the language we use. It has to be language developed with communities, and not thrust upon them. We've seen this over and over in our Community Power and Community Voice programs."[1]

Panelist Vernice Miller-Travis was more passionate in denouncing the word. "Resilience, a word that troubles my soul," she said.

> Because for people of color, resilient means "we are going to keep knocking you down. We are going to flatten you. . .and then we are going to test you and see if you can stand back up." And we do! We keep standing back

up. . . . How about we just do "justice" instead of "resilience"—and stop asking people to get up again and again and again and after a while they cannot get back up? We need to redesign communities and resources to move people out of harm's way. Climate "justice" must not replicate the systemic racial inequities that fueled climate and environmental injustice. We have to think and act differently.—Vernice Miller-Travis

PART II

COMMUNITY ENGAGEMENT, BELONGING, AND POWER

The imperative to engage with our communities is rooted in a deep sense of belonging—they are a part of us, we are a part of them. And belonging, in turn, inspires us to pursue local power as a means of strengthening the places and people that we feel connected to. The two chapters in Part II extend the notion of community to those who may live apart, but share experiences, identities, and traumas. Indigenous people, people with HIV/AIDS, members of other minority groups, and people with histories of involvement in the criminal justice system have all experienced some of the most damaging effects of oppression. But these same populations have also found ways to use their pain as inspiration to pursue change.

Chapter 4, "Confronting Trauma to Change a Community's Health Trajectory," looks at two very different communities that have used the power rooted in historical trauma to confront significant health challenges. In one compelling account, Indigenous people draw on lessons from their ancestors' experience with forced displacement, government brutality, and cultural erasure to fuel their resolve to improve tribal health today. In another, HIV/AIDS activists remain dedicated to ending an epidemic that has taken the lives of millions of people, many of whom long faced stigma and discrimination. Both stories underscore the capacity of united communities to redirect past trauma to positive ends.

Chapter 5, "Harnessing Local Power," illustrates how activists in Austin and Louisiana mobilized low-income residents to claim and exercise their power in the face of daunting obstacles. "How we did it" examples—approaches that forced the city of Austin, Texas, to revise police union contracts and secure access to housing and transportation services, and strategies that upended election outcomes in Louisiana—offer ideas that others can adapt. The chapter concludes with activists' reflections on self-care and the joy that comes from achieving power in partnership with others.

4

Confronting Trauma to Change a Community's Health Trajectory

Gabriel Maldonado, MBA, CEO, TruEvolution

Karina L. Walters, PhD, MSW, Director, Tribal Health Research Office, National Institutes of Health; Former Professor, Co-director, and Principal Investigator, Indigenous Wellness Research Institute at the University of Washington

Disclaimer: *The content of Dr. Walters' presentation is based on work she completed while at the University of Washington and does not represent the official views of the NIH, HHS or the participating academic centers and health systems.*

A community can be defined in many ways, reflecting common culture, religion, geographic location, shared experience, or a combination of these and other attributes. Some communities have existed for centuries, others may be relatively recent in origin. Too often, trauma, with its complex influences on health and well-being, is one of the threads that tie a community together. That trauma might be recent, as it has been for many of the people of New Orleans, or it may have occurred long ago, yet lingers to affect generation after generation.

This chapter tells the story of two communities grappling with the impacts of trauma, past and present. One involves Native people whose health status today reflects the experiences of ancestors who faced genocide at the hands of settlers and a government determined to eradicate them and seize their lands. The other is the LGBTQ+ community, which has historically been ridiculed, excluded, or criminalized, yet found a pathway to come together in the face of the sudden and devastating health crisis that was the HIV/AIDS epidemic. Both narratives reveal the lasting burden of trauma while also highlighting the power that can be uncoiled when a community unites.

Karina Walters, PhD, MSW, is a researcher who directs the National Institutes of Health Tribal Health Research Office and an enrolled member of the Choctaw

Gabriel Maldonado and Karina L. Walters, *Confronting Trauma to Change a Community's Health Trajectory*. In: *Advancing Health Equity for All*. Edited by: Alonzo L. Plough and Thomas A. LaVeist, Oxford University Press. © Robert Wood Johnson Foundation (2026). DOI: 10.1093/9780197809440.003.0004

Nation of Oklahoma. Echoing the experience of many Native tribes in the United States and Canada, her tribe was cast off its ancestral lands by White settlers as the US government pushed ever westward. The damage lingers, but that history of pain has become the springboard for culturally rooted interventions to improve tribal health.

Gabriel Maldonado, MBA, is a long-time grassroots activist committed to improving the lives of LGBTQ+ people, especially people of color. As CEO of TruEvolution, he is part of a determined community response that has challenged the enduring stigma shouldered by this population, which intensified when HIV/AIDS hit in the 1980s. That determination changed the trajectory of the epidemic, and the experience has demonstrated the importance of staying nimble and continuing to engage new leadership to take the movement into the future.

Although the stories of these two communities are rooted in very different cultures and historical experiences, together they help us understand how the experience of trauma can fuel a community's quest for better health.

Applying Lessons from the Ancestors

In April 2023, Karina Walters took the helm of the NIH Tribal Health Research Office, bringing extensive research experience from her previous position as co-director of the Indigenous Wellness Research Institute at the University of Washington School of Social Work. In that capacity, she had developed innovative, culturally credible interventions to address the health inequities plaguing Indigenous communities.

Dr. Walters' work is deeply rooted in her own lived experience as a Choctaw. Guided by what she calls the "original instructions" of her ancestors—the ancient stories and teachings that offer lessons for today—she is committed to helping Native people lead healthier lives and achieve greater well-being. Diverging from mainstream Western methods, she described her approach as "prioritizing our Indigenous framework and bringing in Western tools that might be helpful."

Forced from Land, Home, and Culture

The traditional territories of the Choctaw people spread across what became Louisiana, Mississippi, Alabama, and Tennessee—land that White settlers coveted for their cotton crop. In the winter of 1831, the Choctaw became the first Indian nation to be forced from its land by the federal government. In what came to be called the "Trail of Tears," tribal members trudged on foot to Indian Territory west of the Mississippi River in what is now Oklahoma.

Karina Walters's ancestors walked among them on a journey that killed thousands. In time, tens of thousands of people from other Indian nations were also forced onto the Trail of Tears.

While the federal government had pledged that Indian Territory would remain theirs forever, White settlement continued to expand over time, and Oklahoma was granted statehood in 1907. Indian Territory was gone.

In another forced removal, Native children began to be pushed into boarding schools in 1819, a tragedy that lasted in some places until 1969.[1] During that period, the federal Indian boarding school system operated 408 schools across 37 states and territories, including Alaska and Hawaii, and imposed its own coercive form of education on hundreds of thousands of children. In the hope that they would forget who they were, the children were not allowed to speak their Native language, dress traditionally, or follow Native customs. Abuse of all sorts was common.

Understanding these events requires understanding the mindset of settler colonialism, Dr. Walters believes. While the traditional Indigenous perspective holds, "I am the land, the land is me," settlers insist, "I own the land, the land is mine," a crucial distinction used to justify dispossessing Native people of their territories they have inhabited since time immemorial.

By distorting historical realities, settler colonialism also tried to free future generations from guilt or accountability. "Settler colonialism is about 'erase to replace,'" stresses Dr. Walters. "You erase, and you replace what you erased with—an origin story or a narrative—that supports ongoing settler colonial structures and policies."

> It's about taking the land and erasing us from that land and from the American imagination."—*Karina L. Walters, NIH Tribal Health Research Office*

Brutally forcing a people from their homes to an alien land, and taking children away from their families, tribes, and culture, are stark examples of historical trauma. Walters notes that such collective events strike at the heart of an entire community, combining three assaults: eradicating a people or tribe (genocide); systematically destroying culture, language, and lifeways (ethnocide); and disrupting a people's way of thinking (epistemicide).

Citing her research demonstrating how these past assaults continue to harm the present generation, Dr. Walters believes a purposeful strategy was at play that did three things:

- **"Disrupted our ability to fulfill our original instructions as a people"** by undermining guidance that has passed down for many generations about how to live well and with one another in the natural environment.

- **"Disrupted our relational way of being in this world"** by destabilizing the ways in which people interact with the world around them. The destruction of the buffalo herds on the Great Plains, for example, was a "spiritual assault" that disrupted the relation of Native people to their lands. Before the advent of the White settlers, tens of millions of buffalo roamed the plains. By 1884, fewer than 2,000 remained, destabilizing longstanding rituals and traditions.
- **"Caused us to internalize some of these practices."** When forced into a different culture, as children were in the Indian boarding schools, communities may internalize messages about the cultural superiority of White people that diminish centuries of Native practices and norms.

Native people carry these traumatic experiences with them today, not only in memory, but also quite literally in their bodies. Epigenetic research has documented the biological effects of intergenerational trauma, demonstrating that behavior and environment can affect our genetic profile (see Chapter 6). They alter who we are and how we respond to stress.

Drawing on Historical Trauma

While the generational effects of trauma are undeniable, Dr. Walters believes they can be reframed to become a guiding force for Indigenous people. Drawing on a Native perspective and the insights of Dr. Terry Maresca, a Mohawk elder, Dr. Walters offers the image of water to illustrate the fluidity of this experience:

> Water is "first medicine." We were birthed from our mother's waters. Water is critical to life: our bodies and our earth are mostly comprised of water. Water goes up to the heavens and comes back down. Thus, when one takes a sip of water, one is connected to one's ancestors. And so it is with intergenerational trauma. –Karina Walters, NIH Tribal Health Research Office

Through that lens, people can survive anguishing events, find their way forward, and develop the capacity to thrive. Dr. Walters believes that her ancestors walked the Trail of Tears with a vision of love and life for her, their descendant to come, and she draws power from reconnecting to that vision. Whatever they endured, those who came before her kept looking ahead, filled with care for those who would follow. In her view, nurturing those connections to the past begins with self-care. By tending to her own health, she is not only affecting her own body and family and community but "the next seven generations at least. If I take care of myself, I'm getting the opportunity to correct whatever traumas my ancestors went through, and that is a place of power."

The work with Indigenous tribes that Dr. Walters pursued with her colleagues at the Indigenous Wellness Research Institute followed the three paths described below: developing interventions that reconnect to the original instructions, restoring relational ways of being in the world, and encouraging narrative transformation.

Reconnecting to the Original Instructions

Dr. Walters offers a Choctaw story to demonstrate the relevance of the original instructions from the ancestors:

> Shukvta, also known as Possum, did not watch her children closely, nor did she watch them from the corner of her eyes to make sure they were safe. They wandered off. Bat noticed this and stealthfully swept down and stole Possum's children and took them to live with her in her bat cave. Halambisha, Bat, was sure she could transform Possum's children to be batlike beings living in that cave with her. Possum was frantic, looking everywhere for her children. She encountered Chukfi, Rabbit, who offered to help but was of no use, he made too many blunders. Bat was able to drive him away easily.
>
> Possum wept for she thought her children were lost to her and her People forever. Luksi, Turtle, heard her crying. She went over to help and built a large sacred fire at the entrance to the cave. The smoke drove Bat out of the cave and Luksi walked in and carried all the little possums out on her back. Their tails got singed from the fire and they carry that mark with them to this day. Possum reunited with her children and received instructions from Luksi on how to keep her children close to her and nurture them. Their naked tails are a reminder of how close they came to being transformed into something they are not. Now, Possum always carries her children on her back wherever she goes until it is the right time for them to be on their own. Ome!

This story can be used as a metaphor for healing from the trauma of boarding school. It is a reminder to Indigenous people that their traditional healthful childrearing practices have been healthful, and of the dire consequences to culture and family well-being when outside influences (such as forced relocation to boarding school) try to erase indigeneity.

Importantly, such stories also teach values and practices, showing us here that rekindling sacred fires and teachings allows healing to begin. Although the imprint of trauma—as we see in the possum's now-hairless tail—persists, it serves as a reminder to future generations about the critical importance of healthful childrearing. "Tribes around the world have many such stories that can become building blocks for wellbeing," notes Dr. Walters. "If you look to those original instructions, even children's stories tell us how to live well and healthfully."

Restoring Relational Ways of Being

Respect for one's body, land, and ancestors is fundamental to Native people and so restoring the relational way of being is another key to health. The importance of relational restoration is evident in the value that Native people place on receiving a name. "When you receive a name, you're receiving an understanding of who you are in this world, how you should conduct yourself in the world, how the community should see you, and your responsibilities to that community," explains Dr. Walters.

That tradition can sometimes be used as a form of medicine. For example, people tend to "become their disease" when they talk about behavioral health issues in a way that they don't in the face of physical health challenges. Someone may say, "I am depressed," or "I am an alcoholic," whereas they wouldn't say, "I am cancer," or "I am HIV." Eduardo Duran, PhD, author of *Healing the Soul Wound: Trauma-Informed Counseling for Indigenous Communities,* has explained how Native mental health clinicians can be uniquely sensitive to this. For example, a clinician with connections to the community may press a Native client who declares, "I am depressed" by asking whether he recalls a naming ceremony in which he received the name "depressed." He may also ask his client when depression "visits" him.

This relational way of approaching the problem or dis-ease helps the client become aware that he is not his disease, but rather has a relationship with a disease that causes trouble. As with any relationship, he can change it or learn to manage it, such as by setting limits and boundaries, or breaking ties altogether. "That's the way we incorporate relational restoration into practice," Dr. Walters explains.

Encouraging Narrative Transformation

In a tribal community in the Pacific Northwest, community members were very concerned about the health of their children, half of whom had been diagnosed as obese and at risk of type 2 diabetes. Dr. Walters, who is not a member of their tribe, was engaged to work with them to explore their concerns. In pre-visit archival research, she found photos from the early 1900s of "lean, beautiful, strong, active people," and suspected that historical trauma had played a role in the present-day situation.

Dr. Walters encountered resistance at her first visit, when she was faced with nearly a dozen "grandmas" who were clear they didn't want her to send "any of those White skinny people in here to tell us how to be Indian and what we look like and how we should be, because we've always been big." She was able to turn the conversation around and earn their trust with several carefully phrased questions:

- **"What were your original instructions as a people about food and gathering food and living off the land?"** She knew it was important to start there, rather than asking why their children were obese. The question gave the grandmothers an opening to tell stories about what they were taught about food when they were young.
- **"What disrupted your ability to fulfill your original instructions as a people?"** The grandmothers were clear about this: after being moved to the reservation, they were unable to hunt, fish, garden, or gather wild plants. Many in the tribe refused to use the unfamiliar sacks of flour they were given, suspecting they were poison, and went hungry because they had no access to their traditional foods.
- **"What did your ancestors do to survive so that you are here today?"** This was easy for the group to answer: they always fed the children first, and the biggest children survived. A light bulb went on for everyone—being big was connected to surviving during a famine. "This isn't cultural, this is an historical trauma response," observes Dr. Walters. "It becomes a cultural process over time, but it's not embedded in our original instructions. It was a survival tactic."

  The grandmothers mentioned other survival tactics that might contribute to obesity in the contemporary environment. For example, children learned to eat everything on their plates in boarding school because they didn't know when they would see another meal. Likewise, families might hoard large amounts of food or cook for many more people than they expected at the table as a means of safeguarding against hunger.
- **"Is the same response working for you today?"** The grandmothers agreed that no, it was no longer working, and they now needed healthier approaches to food.

As a result of these conversations, the grandmothers stepped back from a justifiably defensive posture and were able to identify their own strategies for nourishing youth in the contemporary environment. For Dr. Walters, it was another reminder that "how we talk about our story matters. We have an obligation to re-story our lives in healthful ways. My ancestors made a promise to me. In doing that, I'm making a promise to my future generations too."

Dr. Walters calls for interventions that go beyond an individual focus to ones that engage communities, schools, and other societal structures. "You are not going to get population change by focusing only on individual change," she emphasizes. It is important "to find a new narrative by which to understand what the ancestors did to survive and what we can do about that now. This gives us something that we can control today. The environment, the structural conditions must be changed."

Advocating for People with HIV

Another story about trauma, self-care, and determination emerged in another community, at a very different time and place. This one began to unfold in 1981, when a rare disease was first reported in previously healthy young gay men in New York and San Francisco.[2] Soon, it began to be seen in heterosexual injection drug users and, not long after, it became clear that the mysterious illness was also being transmitted through the blood supply. The human immunodeficiency virus (HIV) had arrived, and with it the acquired immunodeficiency syndrome (AIDS), the deadly disease it causes. Millions of people would perish in the coming decades.

Populations that had already been marginalized were actively shunned as infection spread, and the longstanding stigma endured by gay people intensified. Because the disease hit the gay population and people of color hardest, the early government response was muted. President Ronald Reagan famously did not utter the word AIDS in public until September 1985, four years after the epidemic had begun. Senator Jesse Helms introduced a series of legislative amendments in 1987 prohibiting the use of federal funding to provide education about HIV/AIDS. And a school-age child with hemophilia named Ryan White, who had acquired the infection through a blood transfusion, was denied the right to attend school. In these early years, the public responded with more fear and panic than compassion.

By 1994, AIDS had become the leading cause of death for Americans ages 25 to 44.[3] Black people were hit hardest, with a mortality rate in 1998 that was almost 10 times higher than that of White people and three times more than that of Latinos. Entire communities, especially communities of color and those most economically disadvantaged, were devastated as AIDS took the lives of fathers, mothers, partners, children, siblings, friends, and colleagues. Along with the loss of life, people living with AIDS, or surrounded by those facing it, experienced the stigma and discrimination unleashed by the disease and the unnerving uncertainty of who might be next. That trauma has long endured among those who survived.

Nonetheless, activists helped turn back the tide of the epidemic. Unwilling to accept indifference or condemnation, they stepped into the breach, organizing, demonstrating, and lobbying at every level of government in pursuit of more research, new approaches to drug development, broader access to promising therapies, expanded social services, and informed, explicit education about transmission. The availability of new drug therapies in the 1990s resulted in no small part from activists who pushed for significant changes to the system for testing and approving drugs for life-threatening diseases.[4] Determined and creative, they played an outsize role in transforming HIV/AIDS from a death sentence into the chronic disease it is today, which can often be well-managed. Combined with a shifting political climate and accumulating scientific knowledge, they turned trauma into impact.

The federal response evolved slowly, but starting in 2003, every administration was taking aggressive action in some form—until January 20, 2025, when Donald Trump signed an executive order that banned any new government spending on foreign aid projects, which immediately froze all funding for the President's Emergency Plan for AIDS Relief (PEPFAR). PEPFAR, initiated by George W. Bush, had invested $100 billion to combat AIDS across the globe and is credited with saving 25 million lives and preventing millions of new HIV infections. The Obama administration launched the first National HIV/AIDS Strategy in 2010,[5] the first Trump administration spearheaded Ending the HIV Epidemic in 2019 to provide funding in areas with high HIV burdens within the United States,[6] and President Biden updated the National HIV/AIDS Strategy with the goal of ending the HIV epidemic in the United States by 2030.[7]

Significant medical advances accompanied activism and government initiatives, notably pre-exposure prophylaxis (PrEP), which can dramatically reduce the risks of infection resulting from sex or drug use and prevent pregnant women from transmitting HIV to their babies. Anti-retroviral therapies are effective in curbing sexual transmission from someone who is already infected, targeted messaging has made it easier to provide information about sexual health, and innovative delivery strategies have broadened access to therapies. Hope is on the horizon for long-lasting treatments that will limit the need for frequent physician visits. Together, these partners have remapped the path of HIV infection.

The Continuing Threat

Despite all of the medical and technological progress and a greater willingness to have open conversations about sexual health, it is impossible to be sanguine about the course of the HIV/AIDS epidemic. Gabriel Maldonado, a long-time HIV activist, has had a front-row seat for the ever-shifting challenges, especially in communities of color. In 2007, he founded TruEvolution[8] to advocate for health and health equity among Black and Latino LGBTQ+ communities in Riverside, California, part of the vast Inland Empire east of Los Angeles.

That work began at a freighted moment, in the midst of a heated debate over Proposition 8, which added language to the state constitution defining marriage as between a man and a woman, effectively reversing a recent California Supreme Court ruling that same-sex marriage was legal in that state. The statewide proposition passed in November 2008, with 68 percent of Riverside County voting in favor of it. Although same-sex marriages have since been enshrined into federal law, new challenges continue to surface, highlighting the imperative of vigilance and on-the-ground activism.

As the generations that first saw HIV/AIDS emerge fade from the scene, younger representatives in local, state, and federal legislative bodies seem to feel less urgency about championing supportive policies. Other priorities, notably COVID-19, have put new pressures on the public health system, which is already beset by workforce shortages and inadequate resources. The proliferation of misinformation on social media sites and a rising distrust of science add further challenges.

To some degree, early attempts to force people to pay attention to HIV had the unanticipated effect of creating a backlash, given the extent to which many Americans remain uncomfortable with non-heteronormative behavior. "Now we have to pay for the cost of having set off this alarm," says Mr. Maldonado. "Ignorance and anxiety have been part of the conversation from the beginning. People still see HIV and those who have it—as something to be afraid of, to steer away from."

> HIV stigma is not just a fear of HIV itself. It is a combination of morality and sex-based shame and the stigma of being queer or a member of the LGBT community.—*Gabriel Maldonado, TruEvolution*

In today's partisan environment, attempts to normalize HIV prevention and treatment and make it part of routine healthcare have also clashed with ideological biases. In September 2022, a federal judge in Texas ruled that requiring employers to cover medication to curb the spread of HIV violates religious freedom and is unconstitutional.[9] The implications for continued access to the preventive medications that have so altered the course of the epidemic are deeply troubling.

TruEvolution Evolves to Meet Changing Needs

Recognizing the breadth of the social injustices permeating his home region, Mr. Maldonado initially conceived TruEvolution as an advocacy organization. In that role, his team joined with area coalitions to advocate with the city for the needs of homeless, runaway, and street-based LGBTQ+ youth. They also lobbied to change language in the Riverside city charter that referred to "American Negros" and "Orientals," and used only male pronouns, understanding the importance of what he called symbolic tools to ensure that all people feel included in the life of the city.

Over time, TruEvolution evolved into a direct service provider, a change inspired in part by the documentary film about American education, *Waiting for Superman*. The needs of the HIV community were simply too great to "sit around waiting for Superman," realized Mr. Maldonado. Today, TruEvolution is deeply engaged in HIV and sexual health case management, testing and providing linkages to care, behavioral health, youth advocacy and health education, and supportive housing.

Most recently, using its access to at-risk populations, it is developing a partnership with Q Care Plus, a telehealth PrEP delivery system, to broaden access to the tools of prevention. TruEvolution will draw blood and Q Care Plus will provide a telehealth physician visit and deliver PrEP. "It's an innovative way to rapidly expand PrEP delivery and create site-based access," said Mr. Maldonado. "Technology has increased our ability to do both education and service delivery."

Building a Housing Program

In recent years, TruEvolution's involvement in supportive housing has expanded significantly. Initially, the program was one of only a handful of emergency supportive housing providers under Housing Opportunities for Persons with AIDS, the sole federal housing program dedicated to people living with HIV/AIDS. Using a voucher system, TruEvolution's Emergency Housing Program provides 21 days of shelter, along with supportive services that help clients develop a housing plan and budget and search and apply for rentals.

When COVID 19 hit, the organization became a provider for Project Roomkey, a California initiative launched in March 2020 to offer shelter options, such as hotel and motel rooms, to people experiencing homelessness. From there, staff entered into a wider conversation about housing instability and applied for Project Homekey, in partnership with the local housing authority. The state's broader housing program is designed to create permanent or long-term transitional housing options by acquiring or renovating existing structures. TruEvolution is using funds awarded under Project Homekey to support its newest initiative, Project Legacy.

Project Legacy

Project Legacy is a "community campus" that will co-locate housing, social, medical, wellness, and recreational services on a one-acre lot in downtown Riverside. Expected to be completed by the summer of 2023, the campus will include

48 beds, housing mostly people living with HIV or at high risk for infection. Most will be from the LGBTQ+ community, primarily youth, ages 18 through 25, and seniors, ages 65 and older.

Community reaction to Project Legacy has been mixed, reflecting the complicated political makeup of Riverside and neighboring San Bernardino counties. The majority of county residents who once voted for Proposition 8 remain influential, joined by some elected officials who don't want LGBTQ+ populations, or people infected with HIV, living nearby. "There is still a very conservative faction in the region that makes doing social justice work challenging," emphasizes Mr. Maldonado. Bullying and threats against staff have been too common.

Still, "the region is strong and the movement for justice is much more powerful than the status quo," declares Mr. Maldonado. With its distinctive, unifying features, Mr. Maldonado likens it to the Deep South. "We have a way of talking, mannerisms, history, culture," he says. "And we have a respect. If you can maneuver, you can build an allyship across the aisle." The result is a striking degree of collegiality and camaraderie with people in positions of power.

As a result, Project Legacy has received strong support from the private sector, other nonprofits, the city, the county, and the state, which supplemented its Project Homekey award with an additional $10 million grant from its general fund. The process of undertaking a construction project has also opened up access to new revenue streams, previously unknown funders, and government agencies, attracting broad interest in a way that other TruEvolution projects have not.

Encouraging New Approaches to Attract New Leaders

While the organization continues to grow, Mr. Maldonado knows that "as an activist and an advocate, my focus is often on where we are walking backwards." One of his biggest concerns is the stability of the institutions that have helped to transform HIV and the overall continuity of this work. In his years of grassroots HIV activism, Mr. Maldonado has seen many talented leaders exit the field and has yet to see a new generation emerge to take the HIV movement into the future. Organizations still headed by their founders are particularly likely to close when the leader departs, a field-impacting problem that has not been adequately addressed.

Funding is also a constant struggle for small advocacy and service organizations such as TruEvolution. Resources to expand programming are rarely sufficient, and reporting requirements can be difficult for organizations with limited and overworked staff. These constraints in both funding and staff can affect their ability and willingness to pivot and adapt as needs change.

Nonetheless, Mr. Maldonado remains optimistic that community-based organizations engaged with HIV work can be revitalized and "attract new kinds of talent, new kinds of disciplines to add to the HIV movement." He cites his own experience with Project Legacy, which, he says, "inspired me and recommitted me to doing this work." The emergence of nonprofit/for-profit hybrid models, such as social entrepreneurship, a business strategy that aims to have a positive social impact, is another example of a novel approach that could encourage future support and leadership.

A Final Word

As the stories of this chapter illustrate, trauma can impact community health and well-being in many ways. For the Choctaw Nation of Oklahoma, the experience of erasure has filtered through the generations, giving rise to diabetes, obesity, substance abuse, and other poor health outcomes. Yet, as Dr. Walters has shown, this experience can also be the foundation for revitalizing tribal health, allowing people to reconnect to the vision of love and life that their ancestors held onto for them.

For the LGBTQ+ community, the payoff for years of activism has been the reconfiguration of HIV infection into something often preventable or medically manageable. But though the work is not done, the sense of urgency has diminished and new leadership is crucial. It may be time to consider new approaches that resonate with today's young leaders and influencers—the next step in moving past trauma and continuing to change the trajectory of HIV.

Whatever their unique qualities, the work of these very different communities attests to the power of an indomitable spirit, the willingness to do whatever is needed to advance the health of their populations, and the hope for better days ahead that inspires them both.

5

Harnessing Local Power

João Paulo Connolly, Organizing Director, Austin Justice Coalition

Devin Davis, MA, Director of Political Operations, Voters Organized to Educate (New Orleans)

Chris Harris, Policy Director, Austin Justice Coalition
Chas Moore, Executive Director, Austin Justice Coalition

While the experience of trauma contains the seeds for inspired action, as the previous chapter explores, progress also depends on gaining access to power and applying it on behalf of equity and justice. In cities, towns, and rural areas across America, individuals and coalitions are finding ways to seize, exercise, and share that power. Drawing on the inherent strengths of diverse communities, activists and organizers are centering residents in successful efforts to win both short-term victories and longer-term changes in policies and institutions.

They have their work cut out for them. The power-holding deck remains stacked against huge swaths of people in the United States. Those who are not White, lack financial means, or have histories with the criminal justice system regularly confront systems and institutions that devalue their lived experiences and undermine their efforts to promote equitable change. Policies and tactics that enable gerrymandering, exorbitant spending to win elections, and disinformation are effectively tools that reinforce entrenched power structures and maintain inequitable systems that harm communities.

Shifting that power imbalance has become a cornerstone of RWJF's commitment to advancing equity and justice. Engaging with researchers, administrators, and organizers, the Foundation has supported efforts to understand, promote, and spread community power throughout the United States.

This chapter opens with a context-setting framework that examines the nature of community power and some of its underlying principles.

João Paulo Connolly et al., *Harnessing Local Power*. In: *Advancing Health Equity for All*. Edited by: Alonzo L. Plough and Thomas A. LaVeist, Oxford University Press. © Robert Wood Johnson Foundation (2026).
DOI: 10.1093/9780197809440.003.0005

The remaining narrative features models of successes from Austin, Texas, and Louisiana. Concrete examples of "how we did it" highlight victories in increasing police accountability, removing barriers to public housing, securing transportation for unhoused people, and unseating establishment candidates in hotly contested elections.

First, Chas Moore, Chris Harris, and João Paulo Connolly describe their organizing work on behalf of the Austin Justice Coalition, illustrating how outraged but inspired residents alternately dogged and collaborated with officials, inching the city toward equity. Moving eastward to the Orleans Parish in Louisiana, Devin Davis illustrates how an election-winning organizing formula employed by Voters Organized to Educate changed three election outcomes in just two years.

The "boots on the ground" organizing work featured here is constant, intense, and exhausting. Well-funded, state-sanctioned institutions don't change easily, and too many people who benefit from power refuse to cede or even share it. Confronting those entrenched forces are activists who often work in poorly funded organizations alongside low-income residents whose lives are constrained by the imperative of making ends meet. In a nod to this sometimes-overlooked challenge, the chapter closes with contributors' reflections on the importance of self-care, which many of them admit to neglecting at times, and on the profound joy they experience from their work, which drives them forward despite the obstacles.

A Framework for Community Power

Beginning in 2018, RWJF set out to better understand the role of community power in achieving health equity, with the goal of using insights gained to inform its investments. One initiative was "Lead Local: Exploring Community-Driven Change and the Power of Collective Action."[1]

This collaborative research project engaged leaders and practitioners in studies and conversations to "lift up and document how power is built in low-income communities and communities of color, how it shifts over time, the factors that contribute to that shift, and how grassroots organizations do the work to build community power to improve social and economic conditions that advance health, equity, and well-being."[2] Part of the process involved creating a shared definition:

> Community power is the ability of communities most impacted by inequity to act together to voice their needs and hopes for the future and to collectively drive structural change, hold decision-makers accountable, and advance health equity.[3] – *RWJF Lead Local Collaborative*

A core principle of Lead Local is that power is tied to place: "The connection between community-led strategies, place, and health is strong," declares its website. "Research has shown that the people most directly affected by systemic barriers and inequities are the best positioned to drive change in their communities."[4] By speaking powerfully through the lens of their lived experiences, residents have shown themselves to be uniquely effective in driving action. As this chapter illustrates, their stories are as important to securing change as position papers or formal testimony.

Sustaining successful community strategies across time and issue areas is a second tenet of power in the Lead Local framework. The relentless "showing-up" work required to hold onto hard-won victories is sometimes more exhausting than winning them in the first place, yet this is what is required to dismantle inequitable systems and structures.

Small or short-term wins are important on their own terms and perhaps even more useful as stepping stones to longer-term policy changes that can alter governance structures and cultivate new leaders. A report from the collaborative, *Charting a Course for an Equity-Centered Data System,* notes that community power is *instrumental* in changing how governance decisions are made, but it is also "*fundamental* in that it transforms people's ability to see and wield their own power in shaping the systems around them."[5]

Furthermore, as the following vignettes from Austin and Louisiana suggest, power-building strategies that produce wins in one issue area, such as transportation, can be adapted to others, such as healthcare or employment.

Ultimately, health equity cannot exist outside a thriving democracy and a balance of power that affords community residents full agency to steer their course—a third principle of community power. When people come to "see and wield their own power" to effect change, they contribute to building a robust democracy in which diverse voices engage and combine to influence leaders and institutions.

> Although it is individuals who vote . . . it is their combined voices that have the potential to change policies and socioecological condition . . . Democracy plays out through a number of arenas, with the electoral arena being just one. Others include the legislature, judiciary, and administration, all of which can be influenced by organized communities ... – Health Affairs.[6]

Activism, Justice, and Power in Austin

Chas Moore left his home in Houston to attend college in Austin, but his outrage over incidents of explicit racism in Austin and killings across the country at the hands of the police took him on a path away from academia and toward activism.

> I wanted to help people fight in a different way, to give them room to speak up and stand for things in a way that might not be considered respectability politics. – *Chas Moore, Austin Justice Coalition*

Since its co-founding by Mr. Moore and others in 2015, the Austin Justice Coalition[7] has been giving people that room to speak up, organize, and coalesce around an issue. Two principles guide the agency's power-building work.

One is harnessing the energy of residents whose distinct backgrounds and powerful convictions inform a shared vision. After a brief spell as a Washington policy analyst, Chris Harris, the coalition's policy director, returned home to Austin and to advocacy work. "Power is organized money and organized people," he asserts. "We and our constituents can't compete on financial power, but we can marshal the people power."

Working in and with "community" is a second and perhaps more complex principle. "I sometimes think 'community' is really a set of verbs in a trench coat disguised as a noun," says João Paulo Connolly, the organizing director. "It isn't a 'thing' you find, or a place you go to. It doesn't exist without constant actions, rituals, and habits."

The coalition's work to promote police accountability, housing justice, and mobility justice illustrates these principles in actions.

Holding Police Accountable

Traditional attitudes toward public safety allow headline-grabbing incidents of interpersonal violence to stoke fear, leading people to call for zealous law enforcement and carceral responses, Mr. Moore says.

That narrative ignores the things that harm people in far greater numbers—preventable and treatable diseases that disproportionately affect Black and Brown people. "Let's keep people healthy and alive by dealing with the things that are actually killing them," urges Mr. Harris. In his view, ensuring access to healthcare, transportation, housing, and employment is far more likely to reduce interpersonal harms than locking people up.

Agrees Mr. Moore, "It is a little absurd to put someone who has messed up in a cage with a bunch of other people who are also in cages. We deprive them of decent community, lock them up for an extended period, and don't give them the support, love, and affection that everyone needs."

The Austin Justice Coalition had an early opportunity to apply its philosophy after a September 2016 police killing of an unarmed, naked Black teenager shook the city[8] just months before the Austin Police Association contract was due for negotiation. Coalition members believed that making changes in the collective bargaining agreement could add sorely missing transparency and accountability to the city's opaque policing policies.

Organizers and residents became experts in the complicated details of collective bargaining contracts, and they applied that expertise to launch and sustain a relentless high-pressure strategy aimed at bringing community voices to police reform. At its core, the strategy involved packing under-the-radar procedural contract negotiation meetings, which are usually poorly attended, with affected residents. "People don't take selfies at a negotiation meeting," Mr. Moore says, in a nod to the unglamorous and time-consuming investment required.

> Experts without organizing have no power and people who do organizing potentially have power, but not necessarily the authority to get things done on their own. – Chris Harris, Austin Justice Coalition

Activists filled the room at weekly negotiating meetings throughout 2017, took detailed notes, flagged proposed changes to the previous contract, and met with Austin City Council members between formal meetings to press for reform. Failing to have their proposals incorporated into the negotiations, nearly 150 community residents turned out *en masse* at a December city council meeting to protest the terms of the proposed contract, which was due for a vote that night.[9]

Their presence had an impact: The city council rejected the proposal and sent the contract back, asking for a deal that included more transparency, accountability, and funding for mental health and community policing.[10] Unused to having its contract preferences challenged and angered by the turndown, the police association ceased negotiating.

Several months later, a new negotiator for the police association came on board who was far more willing to listen to the activists. Drawing on their input, the city and police association negotiated a new agreement, which was unanimously approved by the city council in November 2018. That contract cost about half of the association's original proposal, with the package of savings reflecting changes in bonuses and stipends, as well as cuts in the ability to cash out accrued time off at retirement.

"Negotiators told us that our presence changed the dynamics of the collective bargaining by compelling real dialogue between the city and the association," wrote Mr. Moore in a co-authored op-ed piece in the *New York Times*.[11]

Highlights from the contract include new policies for the use of body cameras; an end to Class C misdemeanor arrests, such as for traffic violations or public intoxication; changes in use-of-force and de-escalation policies; a new police oversight body allowing anonymous and online complaints; and changes to statutes of limitations and policies that downgraded or expunged records.[12]

Organizers did not get everything they had hoped for, and some of the advances they did make were subsequently watered down. For example, grievances filed by the police association served to dilute the authority of the independent police review board. Armed with the vigilance required to sustain victories, advocates pursued a new strategy, one relying on the electorate, rather than on contract negotiations. They secured a referendum that called for reinstating authority to the review board. After a hard-fought battle, including fending off a counter-referendum backed by the police association, voters overwhelmingly returned authority to the board in May 2023.

> We don't currently have the accountability systems or transparency to ensure compliance with all of the policy changes, but the fact that they are in place has changed some outcomes.– Chris Harris, Austin Justice Coalition

The police department is different, and smaller, than it was five or ten years ago," he added, although he also acknowledged the need for a continuing push to improve oversight.

Organizing for Housing and Mobility Justice on Behalf of Health Equity

When João Paulo Connolly moved to Austin in 2011 from his native Brazil, he found "a lot of energy in the streets, including residual energy from the Occupy Wall Street movement." His activism ultimately led him to become the organizing director of the Austin Justice Coalition.

Two glaring inequities in his chosen city—inadequate housing and poor transportation—caught his attention. "We insist on bringing those two issues together because they are simply not separate," says Mr. Connolly. "Where you live and how you get to the places you need to be are fundamentally connected and have much to do with health equity." As a result of its organizing activities, the coalition has helped to spur policy changes in both housing and transportation.

Promoting Equitable Access to Public Housing

Some of the criteria used by the Housing Authority of the City of Austin to screen potential residents for public housing eligibility were stricter than what was required by federal mandates, especially as they applied to prior involvement with the criminal justice system, according to Mr. Connolly.

For example, the federal Department of Housing and Urban Development prohibits issuing housing vouchers to people convicted of producing methamphetamine on federal property and people on lifetime sex offender registries. Austin's additional restrictions temporarily barred housing applicants convicted of small property crimes, sex work, vandalism, theft, drug possession, and manufacturing or distributing drugs. They also permanently banned people convicted of murder or arson. As a result, about 25 percent of applicants were automatically disqualified.

Starting in late 2021, the coalition organized residents to push for policy changes at every meeting of the housing authority's board. Like the police contract meetings, these had historically generated little interest. That changed when the board received more than 70 letters, including personal stories from individuals returning from prison and letters from a range of Austin advocacy groups. "Meetings are very different when there is an empty room than when there is a room full of folks. So, we gave them headaches, good headaches," chuckles Mr. Connolly.

The organizing worked. In December 2022, the housing authority voted to remove all screening criteria not required by the federal government. This was a two-fold victory, Mr. Connolly notes. "First, people qualify for a voucher they had been denied before. Second, the president of the housing authority publicly affirmed that the authority is not in the criminal justice business and that its job is not to punish, but to provide people access to housing." Putting a human face on the need for housing played a pivotal role in changing policies, the organizers believe.

Securing Free Bus Passes for Unhoused People

Another organizing effort took aim at the need for mobility among unhoused residents. Transportation problems had become a significant source of complaints from individuals who couldn't readily get to their appointments and from service providers forced to divert staff and financial resources to meet increased demand for transportation assistance.

In response, the coalition and others transformed a somewhat ad hoc free bus pass program into a citywide policy that gave unhoused people full access to no-cost bus transportation. An existing program had been "first come, first served, giving people only one or two passes for a specific appointment," explains Mr. Connolly. Continuing its practice of repeatedly showing up at procedural meetings, the coalition organized residents who faithfully attended transit authority meetings through summer 2022 and made sure their voices were heard.

> We organized with the folks experiencing homelessness, who started coming to transit authority board meetings and telling their stories about how bus service was essential for their housing, health, and other needs,
> – João Paulo Connolly, Austin Justice Coalition.

The transit authority responded by distributing bulk passes to agencies that served unhoused populations. "That was a big help, but it was plagued by logistic challenges in getting the passes to the agencies and to the people," Mr. Connolly recalls.

The next goal was to transform that useful but inefficient intervention into an ongoing policy strategy. "We wanted to connect the solution to a broader vision and policy win," Mr. Connolly says. That came in 2023 when the transit system integrated free bus cards for unhoused people into its district-wide conversion to digital passes. The card numbering system tracks the use of free passes, but neither bus operators nor other passengers can see them.

In a promising next step, a pilot program is planned to test the feasibility of linking the passes to the city's homeless management information system, which will allow providers to track medical and social service appointments and address missed appointments sooner. A long-term goal is to learn whether improved transportation access leads to fewer missed appointments and, possibly, to better health outcomes.

Flexing Power to Win Elections in Louisiana

After stints in Arizona and California, Devin Davis came home to New Orleans with a deeper understanding of the intersection of multiple injustices, including anti-immigrant rules, inequitable environmental policies, poverty, and racism. Within that framework, Mr. Davis says that he "found my passion in the liberation of Black and Brown people, work that directly impacts my people."

His early involvement with voting advocacy groups and agencies serving formerly incarcerated people and their families convinced Mr. Davis of the "disconnect between the feelings of those experiencing the impacts of public policies, and the feelings of those who are in power." Determined to eliminate that power imbalance, he now serves as director of political operations for Voters Organized to Educate.[13]

> When people realize they have power, they switch from worry to strategy. It is a beautiful shift when you see people start to believe they can do something. – Devin Davis, Voters Organized to Educate

Founded in 2017, Voters Organized works with and on behalf of formerly and currently incarcerated people and their families. Membership is open to anyone who registers to vote, if they are eligible to do so, attends at least four events each year (e.g., trainings, meetings, or other activities), and volunteers for at least eight hours per year (e.g., canvassing or outreach). Its core strategies are organizing for change, educating people to help them inspire change, promoting progressive candidates for political office, and winning elections.

These strategies have upended three big Louisiana races: district attorney, sheriff, and public service commissioner.

December 2020: A New District Attorney for Orleans Parish

In 2020, the Republican incumbent district attorney of Orleans Parish decided not to run for reelection, leaving the office open for the first time in 12 years. A November primary narrowed the field of candidates to two Democrats: establishment-backed Keva Landrum and progressive Jason Williams. (Most elections in Louisiana require runoffs between the two top vote-getters when no candidate receives 50 percent of the vote in the first round. This means runoffs may involve two candidates from the same party.)

After the primary, Ms. Landrum was in the lead, capturing almost 35 percent of the vote, compared with 29 percent for Mr. Williams. Still, catapulting Mr. Williams into the runoff was considered a major win for progressive forces.

Working with residents, activists developed a criminal justice reform platform and presented it to both candidates. When Mr. Williams pledged his support for the platform, community members hit the streets, blanketing neighborhoods, explaining the issues, telling their stories, and convincing others to turn out to vote. On December 5, 2020, Mr. Williams handily won the run-off with 58 percent of the vote.[14]

December 2021: A New Sheriff for Orleans Parish

The success in the race for district attorney propelled residents to organize the following year to influence the election for sheriff. Marlin Gusman, the 17-year establishment incumbent had been expected to keep his seat, but activists upended that assumption after identifying an alternative, more progressive candidate.

Following the blueprint that put Jason Williams in his seat, they again developed a criminal justice platform, and then sought a candidate to deliver on it. Susan Hutson, the independent police monitor for New Orleans, was highly regarded and supported the platform, but she hadn't considered running for office. "We had to encourage her to enter the race, and it took her some time to build her 'political chops,'" Mr. Davis says.

Despite the learning curve, organizers were impressed with how Ms. Hutson engaged with canvassers and activists, who turned out in massive numbers to share their traumatic interactions with the Orleans Parish prison.

She participated in substantive meetings with residents, listened carefully, and offered thoughtful observations. They, in turn, pushed her campaign into high gear. "After she met with us, we saw a shift in our canvassers and our members," Mr. Davis says. "I have never seen the level of passion that I saw in this race, with young people and older people out on the street, every week, every weekend." On December 11, 2021, Ms. Hutson won with 53 percent of the vote. Both candidates were Democrats.

The significance of these two unexpected victories was not lost on *The Times Picayune/The New Orleans Advocate*, which wrote that "self-styled reformers of the criminal justice system now control New Orleans's two top elected law enforcement posts, a remarkable reversal in a city that was once one of the most incarcerated places on the planet."[15]

December 2022: Reform Comes to the Louisiana Public Service Commission

In still another victory for reformists, Davante Lewis won a hotly contested seat on Louisiana's Public Service Commission in a race that pitted the 30-year-old Democrat against Lambert Boissiere III, an 18-year incumbent who was also a Democrat.

The five-member commission regulates the state's public utilities and sets electricity rates. The commission had been targeted by environmental activists frustrated at its failure to embrace renewable energy and its cozy relationship with utility companies, and by social justice activists angry at its refusal to lower the exorbitant telephone fees imposed on incarcerated people. "The telephone issue struck a big chord with our members because so many people were incurring these costs," Mr. Davis said. Mr. Boissiere had earned the ire of local activists because he had voted against a prior attempt to lower those rates.

Still, it was not easy to organize voters in this contest because positions on the Public Service Commission are not widely discussed. The contest provided an opportunity to demonstrate how much of an impact even a little-known position can have on daily life, and how important it is for residents to understand the systems and structures that govern them. As with the earlier elections, momentum spiked when the progressive candidate reached the run-off. Mr. Lewis won the final election with 59 percent of the vote.[16]

What It Takes

Looking to build power in communities, Voters Organized established a candidate school to prepare local people to run for office, and in early 2023 selected its first cohort. Among the topics: understanding ballot access and political parties, data management, budgeting and grassroots fundraising, public speaking and narrative development, communications and technology, platform development, and ethical leadership. "We don't operate within a political party," emphasizes Mr. Davis. Instead, they look for potential candidates who will push for reforming criminal justice systems. "When a seat becomes available, if there is not a candidate who upholds our values, we will run someone."

To help members sustain their commitment, learn from others, and deepen connections with one another and with their communities, Voters Organized convenes a monthly book club in which participants read and discuss movement-centered books that, as the website explains, "utilize the knowledge of our elders and their written works to mobilize our community to action."[17] The May 2023 book was *We Do This 'Til We Free Us: Abolitionist Organizing and Transformative Justice*, a collection of essays and interviews by Mariame Kala.

In his focused, declarative style, Mr. Davis offers a succinct summary of the strategy that led to three victories in two years:

- collect ideas from people from different backgrounds who believe in a better way;
- let residents speak from their passion, not from talking points;
- turn the ideas and messages into a platform that people believe in;
- turn the platform into a candidate who inspires people to do the work on the ground;
- turn the candidate into a victory; and
- hold the winner accountable.

The Challenge of Self-Care and the Rewards of Activism

Organizing and power-building is hard, relentless work, as the contributors to this chapter know from personal experience. Moments of notable success punctuate long periods of vigilance, attendance at procedural meetings, wading through complex policy and contract documents, and maintaining momentum and morale in the face of daunting obstacles and lost battles.

After an audience member passionately observed, "Your work is exhausting—it is exhausting just to listen to you," the contributors reflected on their efforts to take time for themselves. They don't always succeed, as Mr. Connolly acknowledges by saying that he deserves "a D or D- in self-care." Chris Harris laughingly suggests that his ideal scenario would be to "work myself to burnout, take a month off, rinse, and repeat."

Nonetheless, the contributors all recognize the importance of tending to themselves. "Self-care is an ongoing struggle for me," Devin Davis acknowledges after organizing three elections in less than two years. Scheduling a week off in advance of intense election cycles would be wise, he concludes, mentioning his enthusiasm for hiking and backpacking. Other self-care strategies include spending quality time with partners and friends that does not include work discussions, taking longer breaks from work, and sharing work struggles with colleagues.

The contributors spoke more readily about the joy they take in helping people change their lives and the lives of others. "Meeting people in my community who are more free and have more access to things they need is the most joyful experience," finds Chris Harris.

Agreeing with this, Mr. Connolly mentions the privilege of finding meaning in his work. "It is work, but it is really being in community, forming connections with people who are dreaming together of a new world," he says. His comment seems to resonate widely with others. Adds Devin Davis, "On the spiritual side, I view this as the work of kingdom building and on the physical side, I see it as defining what it means to lead a moral life."

Chas Moore recognizes that even fights that don't yield victories are fights worth having. "I get joy from thinking about the place we haven't been but are working to reach," he says. "When I saw thousands of people at the Capitol fighting for trans rights before a legislature that was not going to listen to them, that brings some joy."

Mr. Connolly agrees, noting, "Even when we don't win, there is a lot of joy in struggling with folks who are like-minded but different."

A Final Word

The intricate concept of community power rests on principles that researchers and academics continue to explore as they expand the knowledge base, engage diverse audiences, and provide tools to help people on the ground. Public discourse and policymaking are increasingly influenced by scholarly literature calling out the interrelationship among community power, equity, and justice.

Equally influential are the activists, organizers, and community residents who continue to push forward, often despite great odds. "Once people—individually or collectively—understand they have power, things seem to move in a way that is just remarkable to me," says Chas Moore. The work of the reformers featured in this chapter offers a roadmap to help others understand and exercise their power in pursuit of social, economic, and health equity.

A key takeaway is that creating opportunities for people of color and people with limited financial means to speak publicly about their lived experiences is an effective way to promote their exercise of power. When formerly incarcerated residents of New Orleans spoke about inhumane treatment in the Orleans

Parish Prison, a new sheriff was elected. When people seeking housing in Austin revealed the hardships imposed by excessive screening criteria, the rules were changed. Although success is not always so immediate, local community residents and agency staff alike are finding their voice, creating and sustaining community with others, and asserting the power that allows meaningful change to endure.

PART III

BUILDING THE HEALTH EQUITY SCAFFOLD

Achieving the ideal of true health equity requires the dedicated attention of clinicians, healthcare systems, community leaders, researchers, and policymakers, supported by the clinical, financial, and data systems that unsdergird the healthcare system in the United States. Systemic racism in American life, with its impact on health status and outcomes, undermines that scaffolding. The contributors to Part III consider new directions to overhaul existing structures so that they provide the necessary support for health equity.

Chapter 6, "The Complex Role of Race in Clinical Decision-making," opens with a look at the significance of the Human Genome Project, which has exposed the myth that there is a genetic basis for race and made explicit the impact of racism on health disparities. Two contributors describe how race is considered in primary care and mental healthcare clinical encounters, and introduce the promise of precision medicine to tailor treatment to genuine individual differences. A focus on kidney disease illustrates the intricacies and implications—for both clinicians and patients—of including race-based data in diagnostic and treatment decisions.

The role of Medicaid as an agent of health equity is examined in Chapter 7, "Leveraging Medicaid to Promote Equity." As the largest single health insurer in the country, Medicaid is a critical source of coverage for millions of people. The chapter opens with a description of the racism that has prevented Medicaid from realizing its full potential and then presents the forward-looking Framework for Health Equity developed by the Centers for Medicare and Medicaid Services. Contributors also showcase multi-part state-level efforts in Louisiana to promote equity under Medicaid and the commitment made by the New Orleans Health Department to promote antiracism both internally and in the larger New Orleans community. *Spotlight: Making the Numbers Work* considers innovative ways to collect, analyze, and share Medicaid data.

Finally, equitable systems for collecting, interpreting, and using health-related data and information are the focus of Chapter 8, "Innovative Research Approaches to Further Health Equity." Building on the idea that researchers must go beyond "methodological canons," contributors present research methods that incorporate systems science to expand understanding of the factors underlying health disparities. The chapter closes with a description of the national collaborative, *Partners for Advancing Health Equity (P4HE)*, designed to foster collaboration, innovation, and knowledge sharing in action-directed research, practice, and policies.

6

The Complex Role of Race in Clinical Decision-making

Vence L. Bonham, JD, Associate Investigator, Social and Behavioral Research Branch, National Human Genome Research Institute, National Institutes of Health

Harold W. Neighbors, PhD, Senior Advisor for Public Health Research and Training, Tulane University Celia Scott Weatherhead School of Public Health and Tropical Medicine; Professor Emeritus, University of Michigan School of Public Health, Center for Research on Ethnicity, Culture and Health, and Program for Research on Black Americans, University of Michigan

Neil R. Powe, MD, MPH, MBA, Chief of Medicine, Zuckerberg San Francisco General Hospital and Trauma Center; Constance B. Wofsy Distinguished Professor and Vice-Chair of Medicine, University of California, San Francisco

Researchers, clinicians, and social justice advocates have long struggled to understand the role that race should play in clinical decision-making. Entrenched beliefs that racial differences have biological implications have been disproven, but differences in health and health outcomes between Black and White people are very real. The lesson learned over time is that these differences are far more likely to be based on generations of discrimination and structural racism than on biological variation. Recognizing that distinction is fundamental to confronting inequities in health and dismantling racist systems of care.

The opening section of this chapter looks at the enduring myth of a genetic basis for race, the role that the Human Genome Project has played in uprooting that belief by establishing that there are essentially no differences across race, and the growing recognition that racism is the true driver of health disparities. Next, Vence L. Bonham, JD, of the National Human Genome Research Institute

Vence L. Bonham et al., *The Complex Role of Race in Clinical Decision-making*. In: *Advancing Health Equity for All*. Edited by: Alonzo L. Plough and Thomas A. LaVeist, Oxford University Press. © Robert Wood Johnson Foundation (2026). DOI: 10.1093/9780197809440.003.0006

(NHGRI) describes recent studies that consider the use of race in primary care encounters and introduces precision medicine as a promising way forward. Tulane University's Harold W. Neighbors, PhD, complements the picture with his look at race as a factor in mental health communication between practitioners and patients.

Then, by looking closely at one serious health problem—chronic kidney disease—Neil R. Powe, MD, MPH, MBA, from the Zuckerberg San Francisco General Hospital and Trauma Center, highlights the complexities of taking race into account in diagnostic and treatment decisions. To close the chapter, Dr. Neighbors, a Black man with chronic kidney disease who was himself harmed by those faulty assumptions, provides a real-world example.

Race as a Social Construct, Racism as a Health Determinant

Two noteworthy advances—one in scientific research and one in racial reckoning—provide a springboard for conversations about the relevance of race in health and healthcare. First, scientific studies have confirmed that the concept of race is socially constructed and has no biological basis. Second, social justice movements have highlighted the role of racism as a determining influence on the health of Black people. Together, this knowledge can help clinicians deliver better healthcare to their patients and inform policymakers and other stakeholders committed to promoting health equity for all.

Biological Basis for Race: Myths and Realities

Convenient myths couched as science once justified both slavery and the brutal treatment of enslaved people.[1] Two especially persistent beliefs—that Black people did not feel pain and that hard work would increase their lung capacity—were endorsed by medical practitioners. Such falsehoods were used not only to rationalize enslavement but also to permit horrific experiments on Black people and to deny them essential treatment and pain relief.

Ultimately, these ideas became ingrained in medical education and clinical practice and linger to this day. In a 2016 study, half of the White medical students and residents surveyed believed one or more race-based fabrications about health. Some thought, for example, that Black skin is thicker than White skin or that Black people have stronger immune systems.[2] Because they rated tolerance for pain as higher among Black patients than among White patients, these future clinicians were more likely to make inaccurate pain treatment decisions and ultimately to deliver suboptimal care.

Despite the endurance of these racist beliefs, the Human Genome Project[3] made it abundantly clear that there is no genetic basis or physiological impact of race. Launched in 1990 at the National Institutes of Health, the Human Genome Project was established to sequence all of the genetic material that makes us human, a goal it accomplished a decade later. When a working draft of the human genome was introduced at a June 2000 White House ceremony, President Bill Clinton declared, "One of the great truths to emerge from this triumphant expedition inside the human genome is that in genetic terms, all human beings, regardless of race, are more than 99.9% the same." And he added, "The most important fact of life on this Earth is our common humanity." Francis Collins, MD, PhD, then director of the NHGRI, reinforced the president's point, saying, "I'm happy that today, the only race we are talking about is the human race."

Racial Differences in Health Outcomes

Recognizing that biology does not explain racial differences in health forces us to look at other historical and continuing forms of race-based oppression, from slavery to Jim Crow, community disinvestment to school segregation, workplace discrimination to criminal justice inequities. Research demonstrates that the chronic stress of dealing with these and other forms of racism on a daily basis causes hormonal reactions that can raise blood pressure, increase heart rate, and build up glucose and fatty acids in the bloodstream, among other effects. Over the years, this continued physiological assault can lead to disease and chronic health conditions, such as heart disease, stroke, and diabetes, a process that noted public health researcher Arline T. Geronimus, ScD, calls "weathering."[4]

The impact is evident in the many studies showing that Blacks and other people of color receive poorer quality healthcare than White people and have poorer health outcomes.[5] Today, Black people in the United States are 60 percent more likely to be diagnosed with diabetes,[6] 50 percent more likely to have a stroke,[7] 30 percent more likely to have high blood pressure,[8] and 30 percent more likely to die from heart disease than non-Hispanic White people. Black people also have the highest death rates for most major cancers and for all cancers combined.[9] The maternal mortality rate for Black women is three times that of non-Hispanic White women, a risk not mitigated by education, income, or access to healthcare.[10]

A complicated mix of factors contributes to these disparities. Neil R. Powe, MD, MPH, MBA, chief of medicine at Zuckerberg San Francisco General Hospital and Trauma Center, offered a framework for considering disease drivers and identifying the most appropriate targets in any pursuit of health equity.[11]

While Dr. Powe focused specifically on kidney disease, the influences outlined here are broadly relevant to any attempt to improve outcomes for people of color:

- **Biology**: Certain gene variants are associated with higher disease risks.
- **Environment**: Poverty, quality of housing, neighborhood stressors, and other factors in a person's living environment contribute to health disparities.
- **Behavior**: Food insecurity and eating practices, physical activity, and relationships with healthcare providers can all impact a person's health.
- **Care delivery**: Lack of access to adequate and appropriate healthcare services is often harmful.
- **Clinical and health policies**: Racism embedded in social and health policies, laws, clinical practice, and culture has far-reaching health effects.

Race and Racism in Clinical Encounters

The distinction between race as a social construct and racism as a health determinant converges in the clinical encounter between patient and physician. When findings from the Human Genome Project were released, geneticists and social scientists began taking a closer look at the value of considering race in medicine. In several provocative articles in *The New England Journal of Medicine* in the early 2000s, some scholars rejected its use altogether while others argued that it merited continuing study.[12] This "storm of conversation" piqued the interest of Vence L. Bonham, JD, associate investigator and director of the Health Disparities Unit in the NHGRI's Social and Behavioral Research Branch, who was already investigating the role of genomics in health disparities. He decided to look more closely at how healthcare professionals consider race.

Beginning in 2009, Mr. Bonham and his team organized a series of focus groups with either Black or White internal medicine physicians, each led by moderators of the same race. They subsequently surveyed physicians on their use of race in clinical practice and what they knew and believed about human genetic variation. The team produced a body of articles that offered insights about how clinical decisions are made.

The research found that both Black and White physicians used race in clinical care decisions, often in similar ways.[13] Both groups recognized, correctly, that the role of genetics in racial health differences is limited, and that other factors, such as access to treatment and quality of care, were more significant determinants. Black physicians, however, were more comfortable talking about social determinants of health and racism than White physicians. Interestingly, physicians who were more anxious in the face of clinical uncertainty were also more likely to use race as a factor in their decision-making compared to physicians who were less anxious, a finding that requires fuller study of the implications.[14]

In what Mr. Bonham considers his seminal work, he and his team developed a scale in 2014 to measure the explicit use of race in making diagnostic and treatment decisions. The Race Attributes in Clinical Evaluation (RACE) scale uses ratings from "none of the time" to "all of the time" as responses to statements such as "I consider my patients' race to better understand their genetic predispositions" and "I consider my patients' race in determining how aggressively to treat particular diseases."[15] The research team has used the RACE scale in surveys with nurse practitioners, nurses, primary care residents, internists, and family medicine physicians to assess the degree to which these health professionals employ race in their clinical decision-making processes.

A separate comparison of nurse practitioners and general internists found that physicians had greater knowledge about how individual genetic variation contributes to different diseases and used race less as a factor in clinical decision-making than nurse practitioners. Investigators indicated the need to examine differences in training and practice that might explain that finding.[16]

They continue to collect data using the RACE scale, and have found that the explicit use of race by primary care practitioners has declined over the past decade.[17] In particular, notes Mr. Bonham, the murder of George Floyd led to "a new look at what was happening around race and racism in our country, and that included medicine." Much of that, he believes, has been led by medical students and residents, who have challenged the appropriateness of using race in medical school curricula.

Individual Variation and Genetic Complexity

As the findings of the Human Genome Project, with its key message of commonality across the human species, become integrated into genetic research, evolving social norms and scientific advances have broadened people's understanding of their own genetic background and ancestral place of origin. This has changed the ways in which people can be identified, hammering still another nail into the coffin of race as a genetic factor in health.

In the 50 years since the Supreme Court's 1967 ruling in *Loving v. Virginia* that interracial marriages are legal, they have increased more than five-fold (from 3 percent to 17 percent).[18] Marriage between people of different races and ethnicities is now a more familiar societal norm, and more individuals identify themselves as multi-racial: 10.2 percent of the population in the 2020 census, up from 2.9 percent in the 2010 census, a 350 percent increase.

The recognition of mixed ancestry has also been propelled by the advent of services such as 23andMe® and Ancestry.com®, which allow anyone willing to submit a saliva sample to learn about their own genetic and ancestral background. The results are often surprising to users. For example, an analysis of 23 and Me users found that the average ancestry of Black users was about 73 percent African and 24 percent European.[19] Such findings make it much less clear what it means to be identified as Black or White.

The current focus on ancestry and ethnicity engendered by these trends has also influenced genetics research. In a review of articles published in *The American Journal of Human Genetics* over 70 years (1949–2018), Mr. Bonham and colleagues found that references to the term "race" in research have decreased substantially, while the use of "ancestry" and "ethnicity" has increased, as has the use of continental labels such as "African," "Asian," and "European."[20] They concluded that these changes suggest "a transition away from the field's history of explicitly biological race science" and noted "a refocusing on racism and race as a social category with biological consequences."

In tandem with that recognition has come greater interest in learning more about genetic variation at the individual level and how that relates to disease risk. Indeed, the emerging field of precision medicine, which can tailor tools of prevention, diagnosis, and treatment to a person's DNA makeup, has elevated its importance. In cancer, for example, it is becoming standard practice to analyze the genetic profile of an individual's tumor in order to custom-tailor treatment.

> We are clearly moving away from making clinical judgments based on a what person looks like or their skin pigment. We're looking more at the individual and their genome to determine the best treatment. –Vence L. Bonham, National Institutes of Health

As precision medicine becomes more integrated into clinical care, it is likely to herald significant clinical improvements. At the same time, access, cost, and knowledge barriers elevate the potential to exacerbate disparities. For example, a major academic research center will have capacities that are not available to poorly resourced local hospitals. Likewise, some providers will be in much stronger positions than others to incorporate precision medicine into their practices. Invariably, these disparities have racist impacts that will need to be addressed if medical advances are to be equitably shared.

How Race Impacts Communication in Mental Healthcare

Issues of race and culture have been a focus of inquiry in the mental health field for decades.[21] There are important clinical parallels between mental and physical health with respect to how racial factors influence the doctor-patient relationship. For social psychologist Harold W. Neighbors, PhD, at Tulane University Celia Scott Weatherhead School of Public Health and Tropical

Medicine, understanding the role of race in treating mental health conditions requires attention to both verbal and non-verbal interpersonal communication.

"Because of the history of enslavement, structural racism, and personal racism, the experiences of people who have different skin pigmentation can be very different, and that means there are cultural differences associated with the differences in the way we look," says Dr. Neighbors. This makes the human tendency to glance at someone and make an immediate judgment about them problematic in communications between patients and clinicians.

All clinical diagnoses depend heavily on that communication. An effective clinical encounter is one in which patients are willing to describe their symptoms and clinicians are able to absorb what they are told. Within this transaction, clinicians "cannot afford to turn away from self-identified racial information, but must try to understand how those experiences have contributed to the symptoms, feelings, and distress that brought the person into mental health counseling," explains Dr. Neighbors.

Where clinicians and patients are racially or ethnically discordant, miscommunication is more likely. "Black patients may not feel comfortable revealing everything right away, and a White clinician may not feel comfortable probing racial issues," he acknowledges.

While the resulting tension is understandable, Dr. Neighbors cautions against a colorblind approach that "tends to avoid the elephant in the room." Clinicians who treat all patients the same "will fall prey to diagnostic mistakes," he feared, especially when standard diagnostic descriptions do not fit the way in which a patient presents. Instead, he said, the clinician has the difficult challenge of deciphering an individual's racial, ethnic, and cultural experience and then adjusting treatment in light of it.

> Issues like race, ethnicity, and culture should be on the table for in spection and definitely not ignored. That's the challenge of clinical medicine.—Harold W. Neighbors, Tulane University Celia Scott Weatherhead School of Public Health and Tropical Medicine

Illustrating the potential for preconceived ideas to lead to incorrect diagnoses or inappropriate treatment, Dr. Neighbors describes a White clinician who inaccurately diagnosed with schizophrenia an incoherently chattering Black patient whose hair was "unruly and matted" and whose behavior was agitated. In fact, the accurate diagnosis should have been bipolar disorder with psychotic features. This fits a fairly common pattern. Dr. Neighbors's research has shown that Black patients are often diagnosed with schizophrenia rather than with a mood disorder, such as depression or bipolar disorder, while White patients are more often diagnosed with a mood disorder.[22] This trend may reflect clinician bias that overemphasizes the relevance of psychotic symptoms rather than mood symptoms in Black patients. This trend is much less evident when clinicians base their diagnoses on transcripts of clinical assessments that do not identify race.[23]

The risk of subjective clinical judgment is that it can allow racial bias to contaminate the mental health diagnostic process. Yet informed clinical judgment is also "the doorway through which adjustments for difference, for race and cultural context, enter the diagnostic and treatment process," stresses Dr. Neighbors. Thus, he believes that effective communication between doctor and patient demands a degree of clinical discretion that must be informed by an understanding of race, racism, and differences in cultural expression.[24]

Rethinking Race-Based Clinical Guidelines

Much like clinician bias, the use of race-based guidelines and algorithms for making diagnostic and treatment decisions can negatively influence medical encounters. Both carry the risk of missing the underlying drivers of racial differences in health outcomes. Yet physicians and other clinicians often rely on disease-specific guidance that has been "corrected" for race, meaning that risk scores on a particular test are adjusted in ways that can influence treatment.

Because racial differences in the health status of large populations most likely reflect the effects of racism, adjusting clinical risk scores on the basis of race does not address the underlying causes of racial disparities. Indeed, it can worsen them. In a recent review, researchers noted that the real key to "making medicine a more antiracist field . . . involves revisiting how clinicians conceptualize race to begin with. One step in this process is reconsidering race correction in order to ensure that our clinical practices do not perpetuate the very inequities we aim to repair."[25]

Race Correction in Kidney Disease Diagnosis: Good Science or Racism?

For almost 50 years, serum creatinine concentration, an indication of the rate at which waste is filtered out of the blood by the kidneys, has been a key factor in evaluating kidney function.[26,27] A 1998 study found that creatinine levels were higher in Black men and women compared to White people at all ages. This finding has been reinforced by multiple studies, though whether this reflects baseline physiological differences or actual differences in kidney function remains unclear.[28] "Black kidney function matters," emphasizes Zuckerberg San Francisco General Hospital's Neil Powe. Black adults in the United States develop end-stage kidney failure three times more often than White adults, and an average of five years earlier.

Serum creatinine levels are one factor in equations used to estimate kidney function in order to determine optimal care. Age, sex, and race are also factored in, and for the past two decades, measures have been adjusted to reflect the research-based differences between Black and White individuals.

In practice, "race correction" has meant that a Black person is considered to have better kidney function than a White person when they have the same creatine levels. Critics have long thought that the use of this race correction has led to poorer care of Black patients with kidney disease because it leads clinicians to assume their kidneys are functioning adequately in situations where they would treat a White patient more aggressively.

Dr. Powe discovered that the race correction does not explain these disparities in diagnosis and treatment. His analysis found that well before the use of race correction equations developed in 1999 and 2009, Black people with chronic kidney disease were referred less frequently to nephologists, which is considered a best practice, and received kidney transplants at lower rates than Whites. "There was this whole fiction that these equations caused these disparities—but these disparities had been around for years," he says. "If all that energy had been put into looking at the real drivers of disparity, we would have made even more progress."

> It's not necessarily biology. It actually might be the social effects that are affecting this biologic variable.—Neil R. Powe, Zuckerberg San Francisco General Hospital and Trauma Center

Nonetheless, the question of whether and how race-related differences in creatine levels should be incorporated into diagnostic testing remained controversial. There is a "tension between ignoring diversity in clinical decisions in order to be race neutral and recognizing differences by race to offer more precise medicine," says Dr. Powe.

Black people do suffer more from end-stage kidney failure, so simply dropping the race correction and using an equation based on White norms for everyone would be discriminatory. Do that, asserts Dr. Powe, and "you're ignoring the data on all the Black people that show this difference. You're saying that we don't need to study Black people because we can study White people and use their value to get Black people to transplant or nephrology referral. You're saying that White is right."

> Providing everyone the same threshold for initiating interventions to address health challenges may represent equality, but giving everyone interventions that they need (i.e., equity) will be far more effective.—Neil R. Powe, Zuckerberg San Francisco General Hospital and Trauma Center[29]

Arguably, eliminating the race correction altogether would confer certain benefits to Black people with kidney disease. By lowering the threshold for establishing problematic kidney function, patients may be able to see a nephrologist more readily, gain a place on the kidney transplant waiting list, and secure more timely access to other treatments.

On the other hand, patients who also have cancer, diabetes, or other diseases could have less access to chemotherapies, pain medications, diabetes drugs, and clinical trials that require minimum standards of kidney function. Given the numbers of people with those diseases, Dr. Powe concluded that the harms of applying White standards would affect millions of Black adults with other diseases, far outweighing potential benefits.[30] In calling for the elimination of the race correction, "people were just thinking about the benefits and were not thinking about the potential harms," he notes. Ultimately, it became clear that a more nuanced consideration of treatment guidelines was called for.

From Race Correction to Health Equity

In 2020, the National Kidney Foundation and the American Society of Nephrology established the Task Force on Reassessing the Inclusion of Race in Diagnosing Kidney Disease. Dr. Powe co-chaired the task force, which drew on evidence and views from pharmacology, clinical chemistry, social sciences, policy, and other fields.

Individuals with chronic kidney disease were included on the task force and contributed an important perspective, raising questions that encouraged other members to focus on the needs of those most affected. "The patients really wanted personalized care," says Dr. Powe. "They wanted their specific factors to be considered in decisions and they didn't want judgmental care."

The result was a recommendation for a new equation that did not include a race correction but did incorporate the higher creatinine levels of Black people into a measure that could be used for patients of all races.[31] Patients on the task force also helped to develop messaging to explain the new equation. "We fixed it in a way that was fair, that didn't ignore the data on Black people, but created a new equation that blends the signal for Black people and the signal for White people," explains Dr. Powe.

A Patient's Experience with the Kidney Disease Race Correction

The real-world implications of the race correction, and the adjustments that were made to it, are evident in the story of Tulane's Harold Neighbors. When he was diagnosed with kidney disease, Dr. Neighbors was startled to learn that beneath the skin his body was considered to be different from that of a White body. "What color are my kidneys? Are my kidneys black?" he asked his physician upon learning that his creatine levels had been "race-corrected," giving him a value four points higher than that of a similar White patient.

After the race correction was eliminated as a result of the task force recommendations, Dr. Neighbors's kidney disease was restaged from 3b to 4. For reference, at stage patients are put on dialysis and become eligible for a transplant.

Going from stage 3b to stage 4 was "an incredible motivational boost to change my behavior," Dr. Neighbors acknowledged. He made a variety of lifestyle changes to manage the disease, avoiding salt, keeping his blood pressure down, controlling his diabetes, exercising, cutting protein intake, and drinking only water. "While these were changes that I had to make irrespective of my race, and the race of my doctor, it raises broader questions regarding possible group differences in making the behavioral changes necessary to manage chronic kidney disease."

Although the underlying biology was unchanged, the message that he had stage 4 disease altered his own approach to self-care and lifestyle as well as some of his clinician's treatment decisions. Dr. Neighbors calls this "co-ownership" of disease management, which is shared between the patient and the doctor. For him, the experience highlighted the need for a deeper understanding of how physicians and patients can work together within a racial context to ensure that acknowledging racial differences helps, rather than harms, clinical decision making.[32] It is also important, he says, to "unravel the mystery of anti-Black implicit bias in the treatment of Black patients by all physicians . . . and to acknowledge the influence of racial history on both the doctor and the patient."

Final Word

As this chapter explains, the sequencing of the human genome proves that people are genetically more alike than not and discredits the idea that there is a biological basis for racial differences in health. At the same time, researchers have consistently documented that Black people have poorer health outcomes and receive lower-quality healthcare than White people.

That means we cannot simply ignore race in medicine or pretend to be colorblind—indeed, doing so means losing the opportunity to understand the many factors that can support health or lead to disease. Nor can we base clinical standards only on the experiences of White people. Instead, we need to recognize the insidious effects of racism and bolster the capacity of clinicians to acknowledge its impact on health in their conversations with patients. As science becomes better able to target treatment based on individual genomic profiles, we will also need to sharpen our capacity to recognize disease markers and develop diagnostic guidelines for diverse groups of people.

In March 2023, the National Academies of Science, Engineering, and Medicine took a crucial stage-setting step in its newly published report, *Using Population Descriptors in Genetics and Genomics Research: A New Framework for an Evolving Field.*[33] Vence Bonham, the lead for the NIH, which sponsored the study, calls it "important for all the conversations that are happening around medicine and race."

The conclusion of the multidisciplinary team is blunt: "Researchers should not use race as a proxy for human genetic variation. In particular, researchers should not assign genetic ancestry group labels to individuals or sets of individuals based on their race, whether self-identified or not." The authors emphasize that racial and ethnic categories, with their origins in social and political history, "make them a poor fit" for understanding human biological diversity.

Recognizing that the multiple environmental factors influencing biological diversity have yet to receive adequate attention, the National Academies has put forward a valuable framework for considering the role of race in clinical decision-making. With that guidance in place, there are new opportunities to conduct scientific investigations through the lens of health equity and to deepen knowledge about the clinical experiences of a diverse range of patients. From there, we can overhaul and strengthen the structures that contribute to better health.

7

Leveraging Medicaid to Promote Equity

Jennifer L. Avegno, MD, MA, Director, New Orleans Health Department and Associate Professor of Emergency Medicine, Louisiana State University, New Orleans

S. Amanda Dumas, MD, MSc, FAAP, Associate Medical Director, Bureau of Health Services Financing (Medicaid), Louisiana Department of Health, and Associate Professor of Clinical Pediatrics, Louisiana State University

In tandem with informed, antiracist clinical decision-making, adequate healthcare coverage is fundamental to equitable health outcomes. The vast Medicaid insurance program, the largest single health insurer in the country, is a pillar here, providing essential services to more than 91 million older adults, individuals with disabilities, and low-income working and unemployed families with children.[1] Medicaid paid for 42 percent of all births[2] and 42 percent of all long-term services and supports in the fiscal year ending September 30, 2020.[3]

During the coronavirus pandemic, enrollment increased by more than 20 million people,[4] but participation is expected to drop precipitously because coverage protections enacted under the 2020 Families First Coronavirus Response Act[5] are expiring. As that decline suggests, certain structural features of Medicaid prevent it from realizing its full potential. Strengthening the program so that it does more to narrow racial disparities and improve health equity has long been a priority of RWJF.

This chapter builds on a summit workshop organized and moderated by Andrew C. Anderson, PhD, assistant professor at Johns Hopkins Bloomberg School of Public Health. It opens with an overview of the inequities and racism that have diluted Medicaid's impact from inception. Next, it introduces the Centers for Medicare and Medicaid Services (CMS) Framework for Health Equity as well as the federal government's "whole government" approach to promoting equity.

Jennifer L. Avegno and S. Amanda Dumas, *Leveraging Medicaid to Promote Equity*. In: *Advancing Health Equity for All*. Edited by: Alonzo L. Plough and Thomas A. LaVeist, Oxford University Press.
 DOI: 10.1093/9780197809440.003.0007

Narrowing the focus, the Louisiana Department of Health's associate medical director, S. Amanda Dumas, describes state-level Medicaid strategies to promote equity. These include inserting equity-focused language in managed care contracts, exercising options available under the Affordable Care Act (ACA), and extending Medicaid postpartum coverage for 12 months, up from just 60 days.

Zooming in further, Jennifer L. Avegno identifies efforts by the New Orleans Health Department, one of only two local health departments in the state, to promote equity and antiracist approaches across the department and in the community. The city's COVID-19 response strategy and its postpartum home visiting program are among its notable accomplishments.

Collecting, analyzing, and sharing Medicaid data was a recurring topic of discussion at the workshop, and this chapter concludes with a Spotlight describing some of the data challenges and the promising, creative initiatives to overcome them.

Medicaid Challenges and Opportunities

Along with its companion Medicare program, Medicaid was one of President Lyndon B. Johnson's landmark Great Society programs of the 1960s. Both were enacted on July 30, 1965, just one month after passage of the Voting Rights Act and less than a year before the Civil Rights Act.[6] After subsequently remaining on the back burner for some years, healthcare returned to a topic of policy focus as the number of uninsured people grew and costs began to escalate. After years of incremental changes, the passage of the highly contested Affordable Care Act in 2010 marked the most significant reform to the healthcare landscape since the 1960s.

Although components of the same legislation, Medicare and Medicaid differ significantly in ways that can foster racial inequities.[7] Unlike Medicare, Medicaid is tied to receipt of public assistance and poverty: "a person had to be poor and fit within a population group deemed worthy of coverage," note researchers from the American Health Law Association.[8] Also unlike Medicare, Medicaid is a partnership in which states share costs with the federal government and have latitude in how they tailor their programs. This arrangement has allowed some states to impose onerous eligibility rules and curtail services and spawned a patchwork of more than 50 Medicaid programs that have historically operated with relatively limited oversight. Further, the program design is skewed toward acute care services provided by physicians in inpatient and outpatient settings, laboratory and x-ray services, and care provided in skilled nursing facilities, rather than preventive or routine care for families with children.

> Over the years, Medicaid has extended significant health coverage and benefits to millions of people, including people of color. Yet, it has often perpetuated disparities and exclusions based on race. – *The Health Law Journal*[9]

Management and coverage improvements over decades have added new categories of coverage, especially for children, and the Affordable Care Act positioned Medicaid to do much more to promote equity and address systemic racism in healthcare. Yet fundamental problems remain.

The Medicaid provisions originally included in the ACA fostered a sense of optimism. In particular, the requirement that the program be offered to nearly all adults under age 65 with incomes below 138 percent of the federal poverty level ($20,120 for an individual in 2023),[10] suggested that large groups of previously uninsured, mostly low-income people would finally gain access to care.

A 2012 Supreme Court decision quashed that hope. While it upheld many provisions of the ACA, the Court's ruling had the practical effect of reducing Medicaid expansion to a state option.[11] As an incentive for states to adopt the expansion, the federal government covers 90 percent of the additional costs.[12] Nonetheless, as of April 2023, 10 states have refused to expand their programs,[13] including seven southern states with large populations of people of color who have historically suffered most from health inequities. Research has found that the likelihood of a state choosing to expand Medicaid "significantly decreases as the percentage of the Black population increases."[14]

In short, the Supreme Court ruling dealt a severe blow to health equity. Researchers, public policymakers, and practitioners continue to struggle to shape a Medicaid program that is equitable and fair. Some of their efforts are described here.

Federal Framework for Promoting Health Equity

Within the federal Department of Health and Human Services, CMS oversees the delivery of health services to more than 170 million people[15] who receive insurance through Medicare, Medicaid, the Children's Health Insurance Program, and the Health Insurance Marketplace.[16]

The 2022 CMS Strategic Framework[17] represents the agency's broad vision and strategies for ensuring that everyone under its purview receives high quality healthcare. "Advance Equity" is the first pillar in the framework, highlighting it as an agency priority. The other pillars, all of which contribute to equity, are "Expand Access," "Engage Partners," "Drive Innovation," "Protect Programs," and "Foster Excellence."

CMS, along with all federal agencies and departments, also operates under a 2021 Executive Order,[18] "Advancing Racial Equity and Support for Underserved Communities through the Federal Government," which established a "whole government" approach to equity and sets a broader context for CMS efforts. Executive Order 13985 asserted that "Affirmatively advancing equity, civil rights, racial justice, and equal opportunity is the responsibility of the whole of our government."

CMS Office of Minority Health

Within CMS, the Office of Minority Health develops and coordinates multiple resources aimed at promoting equity and improving the health of minority populations. It advises all CMS centers on minority health and health disparities, coordinates minority health initiatives within the agency, and conducts research and analyses aimed at eliminating barriers. Key resources of the office are:

- **A Health Equity Data Access Program**[19] that informs the development of culturally and linguistically appropriate interventions.
- **A Framework for Advancing Health Care in Rural, Tribal, and Geographically Isolated Areas**[20] that develops programs and policies to ensure residents in these areas have access to high-quality care, including supporting rural providers.
- **A Minority Research Grant Program**[21] that supports researchers at minority-serving institutions.
- **A Health Equity Technical Assistance Program**[22] that offers coaches and resources to help state agencies and healthcare organizations embed equity in their strategic plans and develop effective means of interacting with individuals, families, and caregivers.

The Office of Minority Health also developed and oversees the CMS *Framework for Health Equity 2022–2032*,[23] a guide for all CMS programs, centers, and offices. The framework incorporates perspectives from stakeholders, research, and other federal efforts, including the CDC's Healthy People[24] initiative. It strives to

> identify and remedy systemic barriers to equity so that every one of the people we serve has a fair and just opportunity to attain their optimal health regardless of race, ethnicity, disability, sexual orientation, gender identity, socioeconomic status, geography, preferred language, or other factors that affect access to care and health outcomes.

The framework's opening statement lays out five priorities:

- expand the collection, reporting, and analysis of standardized data;
- assess causes of disparities within CMS programs and address inequities in policies;
- build capacity of healthcare organizations and the workforce to reduce disparities;
- advance language access, health literacy, and culturally tailored services; and
- increase all forms of accessibility to healthcare services and coverage.

One example of the office's work with state Medicaid agencies is its efforts to encourage all states to implement the newly available option to cover postpartum care for 12 months. Another is supporting states to use their authority to request waivers for demonstration programs aimed at promoting equity.[25]

A closer look at equity activities in Louisiana offers insight on what can be done.

Louisiana's Medicaid Program: An Outlier in the South

Louisiana is home to more than 4.5 million people. Whites comprise 61.6 percent of the state's population, Blacks represent 12.4 percent, and 18.7 percent are Hispanic/Latino, according to US Census estimates, which are based on how people identify themselves.[26] The state's 2021 poverty rate of 19.0 percent is markedly higher than the national rate of 12.3 percent,[27] while median household income is lower ($53,571 compared to a national median of $70,784).[28]

Leveraging Medicaid to Benefit Families with Children

Louisiana has been notable in adopting two equity-promoting and family-friendly Medicaid options.

On January 12, 2016, newly elected governor John Bel Edwards issued an Executive Order[29] directing the state to exercise its option to expand Medicaid coverage under the Affordable Care Act. By December 2022, nearly 770,000 Louisianians were receiving benefits under the expansion program, bringing the total number of beneficiaries to just over two million.[30]

More recently, a provision[31] of the American Rescue Plan Act of 2021 allows states to extend Medicaid coverage for new mothers for 12 months postpartum, or six times longer than the national 60-day coverage requirement. Louisiana added that option to LaMOMS, its Medicaid benefit package for new mothers, effective April 1, 2022, the first day it became available.

Welcome though they are, these initiatives do not go far enough in helping to identify and address the structural racism and health inequity that are intertwined with poverty, according to S. Amanda Dumas of the state health department, who thinks the program can do more.

Early in her career as a pediatrician, a profession she continues to practice, Dr. Dumas learned about her patients' struggles to overcome barriers caused by social and economic inequities, racism, and stigmatization. This led her to explore the intersection of social factors and medicine, and ultimately brought her to the health department, where she devotes 80 percent of her time. She spends the rest as an associate professor of clinical pediatrics at Louisiana State University Health Sciences Center, teaching and mentoring young clinicians. "At the heart of Medicaid's creation is a recognition that there are impoverished people who need healthcare, and I come to work every day with the understanding that we are here to help people who need it," she says.

Yet Medicaid is "a clunky program," Dr. Dumas says, because it was designed to reimburse providers for medically necessary services, as delineated in very specific billable codes. What it failed to capture is the complexity of the "medical necessity" concept. For example, providing donor human milk to premature babies is a life-saving service that allows those babies to reach their full-term weight. Once they do, formula milk is usually suitable, but human milk remains more nutritious. Is donor milk medically necessary? "It is hard to know the point at which a service is no longer the responsibility of the healthcare system," she says. "We have captured a cohort of people who suffer greater health inequity and inequity in general, but it is hard to reduce preventive medicine and social determinants of health into payable units."

Dr. Dumas and her colleagues believe that definitions of medical necessity should be broadened. They are pushing the boundaries of Medicaid regulations, seeking coverage for at least some of the services that "identify and remedy systemic barriers to equity," in accordance with the CMS Framework for Health Equity. One strategy is to establish payment mechanisms that would allow nonprofit agencies to be reimbursed for community health workers and doulas, providers who may lack medical certification but nonetheless deliver essential services to families in their homes and communities. Another strategy entails changing the state's contracts with Medicaid managed care organizations to broaden their responsibilities.

Leveraging Managed Care Contracts on Behalf of Equity

About 90 percent of Louisiana's Medicaid beneficiaries receive their care through one of several managed care organizations under contract to the health department. The Request for Proposals[32] for contracts starting in January 2023 included language requiring those organizations to "specify their health equity strategy, their strategy for population health, and their strategy for integrating physical and behavioral health," Dr. Dumas says.

For example, new language requires each organization to specify the policies, procedures, and initiatives it has in place to promote health equity and how it is "addressing priority social determinants of health, which include aspects of housing, food insecurity, physical safety, and transportation."[33] To ensure that the organizations develop equitable employment practices, the Request for Proposals also requires them to specify their strategies "to recruit, retain, and promote at all levels, personnel and leadership who are representative of the demographic characteristics of its Medicaid managed care population and, in particular, those persons who identify as members of communities underrepresented in the workforce to date."[34]

Other examples of contractual requirements are noted in the data Spotlight at the end of this chapter.

Becoming a More Equitable Health Department

Looking inward, the state health department established initiatives to ensure that its own in-house policies, procedures, and operations advance equity. One component is the Office of Community Partnerships and Health Equity,[35] which has been guiding multidisciplinary Health Equity Action Teams (HEATs) across divisions since January 2019. Following a multifaceted evaluation of HEAT's first phase, the "Health Equity Roadmap Phase 2: Nothing About Us Without Us"[36] was developed to delineate and operationalize equity activities within the department.

The Medicaid HEAT is led by the Quality Section and includes representatives from the eligibility, policy, and program operations and compliance units. Bringing these disparate functions together is beneficial, Dr. Dumas found, because "one person may think about how to use our agency's quality strategy as leverage with the managed care organizations, while someone working in eligibility may think about how to survey beneficiaries about their experiences with the program."

Participation in the HEATs has been challenged by limited staff time and some discomfort among frontline staff used to a traditional top-down bureaucratic structure, where their opinions are not often sought. Dr. Dumas has seen changes in the department, however. "I think equity is being normalized," she says, although more needs to be done.

On the Ground in New Orleans

In her years in the emergency department at a New Orleans safety net hospital, Jennifer Avegno dealt every day with patients struggling to meet basic economic, social, and health needs. "The emergency department is where social determinants of health are on display all the time," she observes.

As director of the New Orleans Health Department since 2018, Dr. Avegno considers the decision to expand Medicaid coverage under the Affordable Care Act "the best thing the state has done in the last eight years." People who had been systematically denied access to care, especially residents of color and people living in poor rural or geographically isolated areas of the state, can now secure health services. "Patients I used to see in the hospital did not have access to primary care or insurance, but now when I ask, the vast majority of them do," she observes.

Benefit coverage does not negate all of Medicaid's shortcomings, however. Stigma, spotty coverage for some conditions, low reimbursement rates that deter providers from accepting Medicaid patients, and inadequate data and analytic resources continue to stymie the system. Moreover, Dr. Avegno agrees with Dr. Dumas that Medicaid will not achieve desirable health outcomes until the social and economic conditions surrounding people's health needs are addressed. "We have opened the door to better access but, that being said, having Medicaid does not guarantee someone the full suite of services," she cautions. "Providing coverage does not undo the generations of structural racism that have kept people of color from attaining levels of success in their lives. It doesn't atone for those sins."

New Orleans Health Department

The New Orleans Health Department,[37] one of only two local health departments in the state, provides and coordinates a range of services for the city's diverse population of just over 375,000 residents, as of July 2021: about one-third are White, almost 60 percent are Black, and about 8 percent are Hispanic/Latino.[38] In March 2023, nearly half of New Orleans residents received Medicaid.[39]

Much of the health department's work focuses on harm reduction, emergency preparedness, environmental health, and other efforts to protect or improve population health. It also operates some direct service programs that serve Medicaid recipients and other low-income residents and carry the promise of reducing inequity and racist structures. These include Women, Infants, and Children (WIC); a health clinic for homeless people; and case management for families with young children.

The state's new Medicaid managed care contracts have been an important step forward in New Orleans. "Those changes put the spotlight on the wraparound services the organizations have to offer Medicaid recipients," says Dr. Avegno. "It got them thinking about social needs and talking to us about programs and partnerships to address them. It was like the lights turned on."

Designing, Testing, Learning

Working in a standalone health department offers Dr. Avegno and her colleagues opportunities to pilot new ideas and collaborate with state officials to address the underlying factors that drive poor health outcomes.

Two such programs are forthcoming in the city. One will provide postpartum home visits to all birthing families in New Orleans. A universal home visiting program, Dr. Avegno believes, can help destigmatize Medicaid and will be a resource for all newborns and their parents. "As a non-Medicaid mother three times over, I would have been overjoyed if someone came to my house in that critical early period," she acknowledges.

The other is a mobile 24/7 crisis unit that will respond to "911" calls in lieu of police when mental health problems are indicated, bringing a public health perspective to crime. "I find a lot of reception to defining crime as a public health crisis and using data to illustrate how crime affects people beyond simply 'how many people did we arrest last week,'" Dr. Avegno says. "Separating mental health emergencies from law enforcement responses allows us to focus on the roots of problems, provide a culturally competent and appropriate response, and address historic inequities in the way communities of color have been treated."

"A Lot of COVID, All the Time"

COVID-19 inevitably dominated the health department for a long stretch. "It was a lot of Covid, all the time," recalls Dr. Avegno. From the outset, the department took forceful action to create an equitable and antiracist response strategy. "That was our mission. We were not going to screw this up."

For example, the department wrested COVID-19 testing sites from federal government operations and ran them itself, deliberately placing sites in areas of historically low access. It continued that practice for vaccines, holding vaccine events in neighborhoods of color and prioritizing residents of color, because they had less access to vaccines and were most vulnerable to the deadly consequences of infection. "If you were a White person living in a wealthy neighborhood, you could drive to Mississippi for your vaccine or call around for sources," Dr. Avegno says, "but you would not get our first vaccine."

An unexpected but welcome side benefit of the COVID-19 experience is greater public understanding and appreciation of the city's health department. "Nobody really knew all that the New Orleans Health Department did before COVID," observes Dr. Avegno. "Now they at least know who we are, and I think for many, we have become a trusted source."

A Final Word

Much about healthcare has changed since the inception of Medicaid in 1965, including incremental attempts to expand coverage, exponential growth in healthcare costs, new awareness of factors that drive health outcomes, and enormous advances in diagnosing and treating acute illnesses. In the context of that evolution, Medicaid remains uniquely positioned to move the country toward new levels of health and well-being.

Despite its challenges and unwieldy structure, it has had an enormous impact on the national coverage landscape: largely because of the Medicaid expansion under the Affordable Care Act, the number of uninsured nonelderly people dropped from 46.5 million in 2010, before passage of the ACA, to 26.7 million in 2014.[40] Many more would be eligible for coverage if their states opted to expand Medicaid benefits. Promoting that expansion remains an important area of emphasis for policymakers, advocates, and academics.

Even universal coverage will not eliminate Medicaid's problematic underpinnings, however. Leverage strategies suggested by the contributors in this chapter, such as making glaringly explicit the connections between social and economic barriers and health outcomes, delineating equity expectations and targets in contracts and collaborations, and assigning adequate resources to generating meaningful and actionable data, show promise. The time is ripe for a full-throated commitment to using Medicaid to advance equity.

Spotlight

Making the Numbers Work

With its data and analytic capacities, Medicaid has the potential to help transform the ways in which healthcare is organized, taking a significant step toward health equity. Unfortunately, the necessary data are hard to come by. Even when they are available, they are difficult to translate into actionable information.

Part of the data problem stems from Medicaid's decentralized structure that allows states discretion in data collection, which in turn makes nationwide aggregation and cross-state comparisons challenging. Other difficulties reflect the limited resources dedicated to cleaning, analyzing, and reporting data in formats useful to policymakers and practitioners.

Throughout their presentations and in conversations with audience participants, summit participants returned to discussions about data challenges and the efforts underway to address them.

Data Challenges

CMS collects Medicaid enrollment data from each state individually. By contrast, it collects Medicare data directly from the Social Security Administration, which eliminates state involvement and enables greater consistency. States differ in the questions they ask Medicaid beneficiaries, how they ask those questions, and how reliably they report the data they do collect. The consequences are apparent in a 2019 CMS examination of state Medicaid data, which deemed race and ethnicity data from five states "unusable" and identified 17 other states as having data of "high concern."[1] These limitations render comparisons across programs difficult and likely distort the healthcare picture across populations.

Amanda Dumas of the Louisiana Department of Health grounds these challenges in state-level experience. Gathering reliable data about living arrangements has been especially difficult, she found, as Medicaid applicants often have insecure housing or live temporarily with extended family in different neighborhoods. In addition, the quality of race and ethnicity data is frequently inadequate because the categories may not fit, or people simply answer "other." Logistical challenges add to the problem. Data obtained from Medicaid enrollment and claims forms are inevitably only as good as the information people provide.

Efforts to understand breastfeeding patterns among Medicaid beneficiaries in Louisiana are illustrative. Gathering reliable information requires developing and adhering to standard protocols, such as establishing who enters the information on a form and when. Is a new mother categorized as "breastfeeding" immediately after the baby is born and the nurse is still in the room to assist with latching? Or 12 hours later, when the exhausted mother asks for formula or is receiving care for complications? Or at some later time, when support from a lactation consultant might have influenced her decision to breastfeed? There are no consistent answers.

Louisiana, like many other states, has limited resources to keep data current, analyze them, and translate them into useful information. "We are often just running to meet the next deadline or meeting a mandated reporting requirement. At some point, we run out of staff power. This leaves some really important questions sitting on the back burner," Dumas says in frustration. The complications of sharing information are a further barrier. "Medicaid is protective of its data and rightly so. It's a lot of responsibility to hand anything out so you want to ensure proper review of its use and be certain that those receiving data understand how to interpret it."

Dr. Dumas anticipates a data crisis as federal Medicaid protections enacted in the midst of COVID-19 are phased out in 2023. Many beneficiaries receiving coverage under those protections have not been subject to periodic case reviews and re-enrollment requirements, and their living, employment, and family circumstances may have changed. "We are going to see a lot of noisy data over the next year," she believes.

Promising Responses

Federal, state, and local officials are trying in various ways to address these kinds of data limitations. In listing data collection and analysis as the first priority in its Health Equity Framework 2022–2032, the CMS Office of Minority Health has elevated the issue throughout the agency. Its November 2022 report, *The Path Forward: Improving Data to Advance Health Equity Solutions*,[2] describes data challenges and initiatives to address them. For example, the agency is prioritizing the collection of data important to understanding health disparities, developing new and unbiased tools and algorithms, and expanding disaggregated data and stratified reporting.

In Louisiana, one response has been the requirement inserted into the state's Medicaid managed care contracts that organizations assess the health needs of every enrollee, and report on their clinical status, housing arrangements, and other social determinates. The contracts also require managed care providers to describe how they will "stratify, analyze, and act on data regarding inequities in care."[3]

Another approach comes from the New Orleans Health Department, which tapped into the analytic resources of its in-house homeland security team to inform its crisis response to COVID-19. "We gave the team more than 10,000 addresses of people who had gone to the first New Orleans COVID-19 testing sites," Dr. Avegno says. The map created by the team "glaringly identified areas where people could not access tests, and not surprisingly, these were the areas of highest social vulnerability," she adds. The department put its testing sites in those areas and later established vaccine sites there, too. "We didn't have access to great data and certainly not standardized data, but we were able to take what we had, turn it on its head, and keep refining it," Dr. Avegno concludes.

8

Innovative Research Approaches to Further Health Equity

Gail Christopher, DN, Executive Director, National Collaborative for Health Equity

Irene Headen, PhD, MS, Assistant Professor of Black Health, Drexel University Dornsife School of Public Health

Thomas A. LaVeist, PhD, Dean and Weatherhead Chair, Tulane University Celia Scott Weatherhead School of Public Health and Tropical Medicine

Alonzo L. Plough, PhD, MA, MPH, Vice President, Research-Evaluation-Learning, and Chief Science Officer, Robert Wood Johnson Foundation

Kristefer Stojanovski, PhD, MPH, Research Assistant Professor, Tulane University Celia Scott Weatherhead School of Public Health and Tropical Medicine; Research Director, Partners for Advancing Health Equity

The clinical and policy approaches described in this section depend heavily on evidence that enlightens and guides actions designed to generate greater health equity. But research that does not consider the lived experiences of all relevant stakeholders, or is biased in its overarching approach, can reinforce stereotypes and often support ideas that selectively benefit the privileged. This final chapter explores innovative methodologies and models for collecting, interpreting, and using data in new ways to support health equity.

In the chapter's opening section, Alonzo L. Plough, vice president, Research-Evaluation-Learning at the Robert Wood Johnson Foundation, and Thomas A. LaVeist, dean of Tulane University Celia Scott Weatherhead School of Public Health and Tropical Medicine, consider opportunities to go beyond

Gail Christopher et al., *Innovative Research Approaches to Further Health Equity*. In: *Advancing Health Equity for All*. Edited by: Alonzo L. Plough and Thomas A. LaVeist, Oxford University Press. © Robert Wood Johnson Foundation (2026). DOI: 10.1093/9780197809440.003.0008 academic convention so that health equity has a more prominent place in the research agenda.

Next, Gail Christopher, DN, executive director of the National Collaborative for Health Equity, describes the Truth, Racial Healing & Transformation™ (TRHT™) framework. TRHT is a comprehensive framework with five interconnected pillars on which to organize, undergird, and unite efforts to end racism.

Two scholars then highlight research methods based on systems science. Kristefer Stojanovski, research assistant professor at Tulane University Celia Scott Weatherhead School of Public Health and Tropical Medicine, describes techniques for using complex systems theory to investigate HIV risk and how to think in systems. Community-based system dynamics, a type of group model building, centers the work of Irene Headen, assistant professor of Black health at Drexel Dornsife School of Public Health, who explores the connections between neighborhood factors and Black maternal and child health.

Finally, Dr. LaVeist closes the chapter by describing Partners for Advancing Health Equity (P4HE), a national collaborative led by Tulane and funded by RWJF. P4HE is designed, he says, "to spark discussion, share learning, foster collaboration, and facilitate resource exchange for the promotion of action-oriented health equity research, practice, and policies."

Beyond Methodological Canons

The profound impact of racism on health, coupled with the weaknesses of the public health system that became shockingly apparent during the COVID-19 pandemic, represents a call to action for transforming public health research. To have the urgently needed effect, researchers and the health data infrastructure they depend on must transcend what RWJF's Alonzo L. Plough calls "methodological canons"—that is, the unquestioned practices that have long governed how research is conducted.

Reimagining Data in Pursuit of Health Equity

Understanding structural racism and the threat it poses to public health requires that we interrogate conventional approaches to constructing and defining data. That process begins by engaging in innovative, community-led knowledge building.

To "reimagine how data are collected, shared, and used, and to identify the investments needed to improve health equity," RWJF established the

National Commission to Transform Public Health Data Systems, led by Dr. Gail Christopher, in 2021. In its report, *Charting a Course for an Equity-Centered Data System*,[1] the commission issued recommendations targeted at stakeholders as varied as public health, healthcare systems, academia and research institutions, philanthropy, businesses, nonprofits, professional associations, and government at all levels.[2]

The commission's overarching recommendation was to "Ensure public health measurement captures and addresses structural racism and other inequities." With that statement, Dr. Plough says that the commission posed a "challenge to the conventional constructs that researchers were trained in" and underscored the need for new approaches to knowledge building. Its message is that academia, which has traditionally operated in relative isolation, cannot be the only place where knowledge is formalized and validated. Local and regional partnerships are also essential to allow innovations to take hold and foster greater trust and transparency in decision-making, notes Dr. Plough. At their best, such partnerships can help to grow cross-sector collaborations and authentic community engagement, disseminate wellbeing metrics, disaggregate community-level data to sharpen insights about diverse populations, and promote social justice movements and explicit antiracist activism.

Dr. Plough describes several RWJF initiatives that focus on developing equitable data and addressing structural racism as a public health problem in new ways:

- A collaboration with the Centers for Disease Control and Prevention (CDC) Foundation uses PLACES[3] health data in five communities across the country to design innovative solutions that consider the social and structural factors affecting local health outcomes.
- A network of Historically Black Colleges and Universities (HBCUs) in the Gulf region[4] is working to bring the climate and environmental justice movement more deeply into the public health practices of the Gulf states. RWJF's support amplifies a 25-year grant from the 2010 BP oil spill settlement to the Gulf Research Program of the National Academy of Sciences.
- The Modernized Anti-Racist Data Ecosystems (MADE) for Health Justice[5] project, administered by the de Beaumont Foundation, is accelerating the development of health-focused local data ecosystems centered on antiracism, equity, justice, and community power. The program has generated a great deal of interest among local organizations that "want to be a part of having actionable data to improve health and wellbeing in their communities," says Dr. Plough.

New Guidelines for Gathering Actionable Evidence

To change the traditional frameworks of research and data collection, Dr. Plough and Tulane's Thomas A. LaVeist offered the following recommendations to the leaders of research institutions:

- **Investigate across disciplines**. Traditionally, researchers have been "trained to think that problems occur within disciplines," says Dr. Plough. The truth is they do not, but the academic system seldom offers the transdisciplinary training scholars need to address issues like health equity and structural racism. Adds Dr. LaVeist, "People in academic positions of power must value this and develop programs that cut across disciplines."
- **Develop strong partnerships with communities**. "Universities need to see themselves as partners with the community and understand that the community is an authentic partner that the university can learn from and work collaboratively with," advises Dr. Plough. That framing can then strengthen the necessary partnerships between the academic and field practice sides of health.
- **Strive for community-led research**. Ideally, when undertaking community-based participatory research, the community should be the leader, particularly in defining the problems to be studied.
- **Support a diverse range of researchers**. Mentorship, access to financial resources, and opportunities for professional and network growth all support the career development of underrepresented researchers (see RWJF's Health Equity Scholars for Action[6] and Health Policy Research Scholars[7] as examples).
- **Increase the scope of faculty reward systems**. Faculty involvement in innovative, community-based participatory research should be valued, recognized, and included in tenure decisions and other mechanisms used to reward faculty members.
- **Use the power of academic position**. More people with a deep commitment to equity are needed in academic leadership positions, including at the dean and department chair levels. Their influence and the resources they control can shape equity-focused research agendas, further transdisciplinary investigation, and expand reward and incentive systems.
- **Ensure that the university itself contributes to equity**. In many communities, universities are the largest employers and the ones that do the most business with other businesses. "The impact that we can have is so much bigger than just the impact we have on our students," says Dr. LaVeist. Among the tools at their disposal, universities can pay a living wage, provide a comprehensive benefits package, and support minority-owned businesses. One example

is Dr. LaVeist's success at persuading Tulane to open an account with the New Orleans-based Liberty Bank, the largest Black-owned bank in the country.

Truth, Racial Healing & Transformation™: A Framework for Communities and Research

Gail Christopher of the National Collaborative for Health Equity is as convinced as Drs. Plough and LaVeist that health equity cannot be achieved without ending racism. Rooted in what she calls a "hierarchy of human value," racism has been one of the grounding features of United States history, yet the nation has never faced its racist past. (Dr. Christopher's analysis of racial hierarchy is described more fully in "Racial Hierarchy, Race Narrative, and the Structures that Sustain Them," a chapter in volume 6 of RWJF's Culture of Health Series, *Necessary Conversations: Understanding Racism as a Barrier to Achieving Health Equity*[8].)

In a quest for the kind of dedicated truth process that South Africa and other nations have employed, Dr. Christopher created the Truth, Racial Health & Transformation[9]™ (TRHT) framework in her previous capacity as senior advisor and vice president at the W.K. Kellogg Foundation. TRHT is a community-based model for addressing the historic and contemporary effects of racism in communities and institutions so that transformational and sustainable change can occur. "[TRHT communities] work to replace the deeply held belief system that fuels racism with one that sees the inherent value of all people."[10]

The framework encompasses five pillars: two foundational areas that all TRHT communities should address and three action areas that communities can choose to pursue singly or in combination with one another. Each pillar offers ample opportunity for equity-centered research and a structure for pursuing systems change. Dr. Christopher calls on researchers to ensure that a vision of equitable health, well-being, and democracy drives the work forward.

Two Foundational Pillars for All TRHT Communities

Two foundational pillars, each critical for transformation, support each other; together, they are greater than the sum of their parts.

Narrative Change: Truth Telling

Because belief systems are driven by the stories that people pass along over time, false narratives can damage our understanding of the world and our relationships within it. To foster what Dr. Christopher labels "change for equity," she believes that news media, school curricula, digital media, cultural and educational institutions, and other disseminators of information must offer fuller and more authentic narratives. In short, they must tell the truth.

Describing the potential of social media and the algorithms that drive it to polarize and divide society as a "runaway train," Dr. Christopher called for research to unpack both the benefits and threats of today's media. She also emphasized the need to disseminate research results to those in power at the local, state, and federal levels in order to "leverage the potential of social media to foster community, unity, dialogue, and discourse that would actually be healing for the country."

Racial Healing: Trust and Relationship Building

This second pillar of TRHT focuses on bringing communities together by centering equity in the work of building mutually respectful relationships. The goal is to honor and value individual and common humanity in ways that strengthen connections across racial and ethnic lines, between generations, and among diverse communities. A fertile area for research in this domain is exploring how a community can gain greater agency in defining and shaping its own data to accurately represent itself as it builds relationships among its constituents and with other communities.

The two foundational pillars of narrative change and relationship building are strongly connected, Dr. Christopher emphasizes. "There's actually something very healing in the process of sharing your story and being listened to sincerely." The capacity to map and measure relationships, networks, and connections among people allows pre-existing and emerging connections and relationships to be tracked and linked to indicators for opportunity, community investment, and change. Local TRHT communities are learning how to innovate in this way, and it is a promising area for further research.

Three Pillars of Community Action

The TRHT framework suggests three avenues for exploring and correcting the destructive concept of racial hierarchy that is embedded in society: separation, law, and the economy.

Separation: Segregation, Colonization, and Concentrated Poverty

The "long, long legacy of division and isolation in the structure of our communities," says Dr. Christopher, was a deliberate strategy to maintain racial hierarchy. Redlining, a government-sanctioned process of dividing communities based on undocumented differences in investment risk, is only one of many tools that were used to keep people apart (see Chapter 2).

To gain a deeper understanding of the enduring consequences, Dr. Christopher calls on researchers to consider "those ways in which enforced separation and segregation have produced a legacy that creates an opportunity for real investment and real change." This is a timely moment for doing so, given the momentum to tackle racism that is apparent at all levels of government. In line with the Biden Administration's priorities, every federal agency has crafted a plan for achieving equity in its policy and programming. Likewise, more than 250 state and local public health agencies and departments have declared racism a public health crisis, giving communities a unique opportunity to define the research questions that can inform action. "We must seize this unprecedented moment when an intention is being expressed directly about achieving equity and provide the research to help catapult and mobilize the work that is needed," says Dr. Christopher.

Law: Civil, Criminal, and Public Policies

The legal system offers numerous opportunities for research that can inform a vision of equity. The starting place, says Dr. Christopher, is recognizing that "the legal system in this country was designed to maintain this false hierarchy of human value." She identified three areas of law that are particularly ripe for study: voting, criminal justice, and immigration.

Voting, she says, is "the most important aspect of our legal system, both in terms of the opportunity for achieving and sustaining equity, but also in terms of the viability of our democracy." She urges the research community to explore inequitable access to voting, and especially to analyze ways to encourage more young people to vote.

The criminal justice system can be another locus of innovative research. The TRHT calls for a deeper understanding of discriminatory civil and criminal laws and the policies that emanate from them, as well as an exploration of what public safety means and the social determinants that influence it. The lack of adequate and consistent data is a challenge to advancing a body of knowledge here.

The vast challenges of immigration policy also demand attention. Given the current political climate, there is an urgent need for detailed and nuanced research and data that can inform a just policy agenda at the local, state, and federal levels. The authentic voices of the most affected communities must be front and center of new thinking.

Economy: Structured Inequality and Barriers to Opportunity

In Dr. Christopher's view, racism has driven an economy that is unfair, unjust, and inequitable. "We need to be focused on the harm that these widening wealth divides are causing, and we need to do research that documents the power of intervention," she urges.

One strategy that has already shown benefits and merits further scrutiny is a guaranteed minimum income for all. For example, research demonstrates that pregnant women who receive unrestricted income have better birth outcomes.[11] Likewise, the 2021 expansion of the Child Tax Credit reduced the rate of child poverty by a dramatic 44 percent.[12]

An Equity-Centered Research Agenda

To have a truly equity-centered research agenda, researchers must stop "romancing the problems and merely documenting the inequities and, rather, be driven by a clear set of expectations for progress," insists Dr. Christopher.

She cites the Health Opportunity and Equity (HOPE) Initiative[13] led by the National Collaborative for Health Equity, which lays out a concrete set of action steps.[14] To guide decisions, the HOPE data track 27 indicators (such as adult and child health status, food security, and affordable housing), grouped in five domains (health outcomes, social and economic factors, community and safety factors, physical environment, and access to healthcare). These indicators are tracked by race, ethnicity, and socioeconomic status, and are available for all 50 states and the District of Columbia.

The HOPE data tool includes a distance-to-goal measure that shows how much progress the nation and each state must make to achieve the HOPE goal on each indicator, both overall and by race and ethnicity.

"The expectation is that we're going to provide the opportunities for people to be healthy," says Dr. Christopher. By centering equity, "we can design innovative interventions, strategies, and research projects that are driven by an understanding of the primacy of changing our hearts and our minds and committing to creating a future that values all people equally."

Using Systems Science to Further Health Equity

The factors that undergird structural racism and lead to health disparities and inequity do not operate in isolation. Rather, it is the interactions among those factors that give rise to persistent injustice. That means traditional methodologies that focus primarily on the impact of individual and interpersonal determinants are inadequate for the crucial task of understanding how racism threatens public health. Expansive thinking that moves beyond conventional methods and approaches is critical to be able to grapple fully with the challenges.

Systems science originated in engineering and business as a way to model the complex and interrelated factors that generate a particular behavior. By modeling the intricacy of systems in which people live, work, learn, and play, systems science allows the many influences on health and well-being to be studied more comprehensively.[15] Focusing on the multiple elements of a system, how they interact, and the effects that emerge creates an opportunity to direct attention upstream to the broader societal determinants of disparate health pathways. Systems science can help "connect the dots" across policies, interpersonal behavior, and past and current laws to allow for a more nuanced understanding of structural racism.

Among the principles that are key to systems thinking:[16]

- **Purpose**. Each system is structured to work toward an intended purpose although a system will evolve in its own way in practice, sometimes leading to an unanticipated place or outcome.
- **Feedback**. A system is dynamic, not static, with its many elements interacting through feedback loops that either amplify or counteract behaviors within the system.
- **Adaptation**. Systems adapt in response to new conditions and information.
- **Emergence**. A system is not merely the sum of its parts but, rather, the cumulative effect of its many interactions, feedback loops, adaptation, and evolution. This collective behavior is a crucial aspect of systems thinking.

In recent years, systems thinking has been gaining traction in the study of health equity,[17] but adding systems science tools to the health equity toolbox can still require a bit of case-selling. Two early-career researchers are enthusiastically making that case, exploring how systems science theories, methods, techniques, and analyses can be used in more comprehensive investigations of health inequities.

Putting Systems Science to Work in HIV Research

"It is important to unpack the systems that perpetuate health inequities," says Kristefer Stojanovski, research assistant professor at the Tulane University Celia Scott Weatherhead School of Public Health and Tropical Medicine, who is using systems science to research the risks of HIV infection. "Researchers like to put things in boxes and study how one box relates to another as if these were linear processes. In fact, there is all this messiness behind the scenes.". "Systems science offers us a strategy, a framework to pull apart these systems so we can understand how racism—as a system—shapes health inequities and creates poor health among Black persons."—*Kristefer Stojanovski, Tulane University Celia Scott Weatherhead School of Public Health and Tropical Medicine*

Individual risk factors for HIV infection are well known and include unreliable use of condoms, multiple sex partners, and needle-sharing among injection drug users. None of these behaviors operates in a vacuum, however; all are part of an interlaced web that also includes policies, laws, and other upstream influences. A system at work is evident in data showing that a pattern of recent HIV infections among people in the same social network increases the risk for everyone within that network.[18] Likewise, risk is lower in a social network that includes more people who are HIV-negative or who use pre-exposure prophylaxis (PrEP). System influences are also evident in findings that education, access, and affordability affect condom use and that PrEP use can be altered by policies broadening healthcare and health insurance coverage.

By de-siloing the factors associated with HIV risk, "systems science attempts to study all of these factors at the same time," says Dr. Stojanovski. His research has found that in countries where less stigma is associated with sexual behavior and legal protections are in place for gay and bisexual men, rates of HIV infection are lower compared to countries without such norms or protections.[19] For example, a person who has had sex with 51 or more partners without using a condom in the past year, while still at high risk for HIV, is 20 percent less likely to become infected if they live in a country that protects LGBTQ+ individuals.

"How is it that someone can conduct the same risky behavior in different contexts and have a different risk of infection?" asks Dr. Stojanovski. In search of an answer, he reframed the research question he was exploring from "what are the predictors of HIV diagnosis?" to "how does the policy context predict HIV diagnosis?"

Policies that stigmatize the LGBTQ+ population also harm mental health, which can then affect both sexual behavior, including number of partners and condom use, and compliance with prevention or treatment regimens. "So, there are structural factors shaping HIV risk," says Dr. Stojanovski. "This is where systems science can be helpful."

Systems Science Methods

The following tools, described here by Dr. Stojanovski in the context of HIV research, use system science to leverage an existing evidence base.

Evidence synthesis is an approach to connecting findings from multiple studies and disciplines. Artificial intelligence can play a role here. Dr. Stojanovski has used ChatGPT to extract relevant pieces of data and information from a set of research articles, allowing him to aggregate and analyze findings much more quickly than if he had to comb through them article by article. Software, such as Covidence,[20] can also help to automate the process of synthesizing evidence.

Systems mapping can highlight connections by creating visual representations of the interactions among different elements of a system. Systems mapping software, such as Kumu,[21] which is free and available online, enables researchers to visualize and tease out complex relationships. Higher-order factors, such as a country's gay rights legislation, can be incorporated into a model that also includes individual behavioral risk factors.

In agent-based modeling, simulated "agents" (that is, people) are put into artificially constructed environments that have rules, such as stigmatizing LGBTQ+ policies, which can influence other parts of the system. Varying the parameters in the model can shed light on the disparities in HIV infection rates between Black and White gay men. Cluster computers can run simulations millions of times, generating data and questions that a researcher can then use as the basis for a real-world study.

An example is the intersection of PrEP prescriptions, individual behavior, and race. Research indicates that Black gay men in the United States are more likely to use condoms, less likely to use drugs, and have fewer sex partners than White gay men.[22] "Everything Black gay men are doing at the individual level is more protective than what White gay men are doing," explains Dr. Stojanovski. "Yet they still have the highest risk for HIV."

Part of the explanation is that Black gay men are not prescribed PrEP as often as White men, increasing their personal risk and the risk to their social networks and the population of Black gay men. This is exacerbated by the higher probability of adverse health outcomes that already confront Black people for a host of reasons linked by racism (see Chapter 6).

Agent-based modeling allows the rate of PrEP prescription to be varied to learn how best to drive change. Sometimes, the results are startling. For example, one agent-based study found that prescribing PrEP at equal rates to Black and White agents *increased* the disparity in HIV infections.[23] While HIV infection rates decreased in both groups, the decrease for Black agents was significantly less than that for White agents, widening the racial gap. This outcome likely reflects inequities associated with barriers of access, such as cost and availability, and with stigma, such as concerns and misconceptions about PrEP, which reduce medication uptake.

"This is where equity comes in," Dr. Stojanovski explains. "Just because you prescribe equally doesn't mean you have addressed the underlying disparity in the health of Black and White people due to racism." Achieving health equity in this case requires addressing barriers to uptake.

Dr. Stojanovski notes that increasing the rate of PrEP use among Black men would likely lower overall societal risk for HIV—an example of emergence, the collective behavior of the system. "If we want to understand larger issues and how they impact people at the individual level, then we need to start studying neighborhoods, organizations, social circles, communities, and the interaction across all of those," he says. "That's where systems science methods come in."

Community-Based System Dynamics

Irene Headen, assistant professor of Black health at Drexel University Dornsife School of Public Health, studies Black maternal health and is especially interested in how multiple elements of the neighborhood environment, such as housing, food, and transportation, interact to affect the experience of pregnancy and perpetuate inequities in birth outcomes. She was drawn to systems science as a way to incorporate these multiple elements and develop evidence based on local experience that could drive more effective action.

Traditional research methods focus on identifying linear relationships, such as between socioeconomic status and adverse birth outcomes, or between food security and adverse birth outcomes. Systems science is appealing, she explained, because it acknowledges these individual contributors but can also uncover the multiplicative effect of several factors operating at the same time. That provides an opportunity to better answer questions such as: To what extent does adequate access to food protect against adverse birth outcomes in an under-resourced environment?

"The ability to capture these interactions and interdependent relationships matters," Dr. Headen stresses. "It is hard to understand the ecosystem of structural racism and how it produces inequitable environments if we isolate the impacts of racist policies within these different domains."

> Institutional racism within the job environment interacts with institutional racism within the housing environment, which interacts with institutional racism within the education environment. –Irene Headen, Drexel Dornsife School of Public Health

A Focus on Community Ownership and Control

The use of systems science to drive health equity requires researchers to engage multiple stakeholders in defining the research questions of concern, mapping the system creating undesirable outcomes, and translating findings into action. Certainly, policymakers and decision makers who understand how a system works, how different parties use that system, and what drives their assumptions about change belong in the mix. For example, providers should be included in an examination of racism in a clinical obstetrics setting.

However, seating community members "who are experiencing the brunt of systems of structural oppression at the table" is absolutely central, stresses Dr. Headen. In the example of maternal health, community members tend to be the least heard part of the system. "For problems of structural exclusion and marginalization, centering the voices and experiences of those who are most in the margins remains integral to correctly operationalizing the problem at hand," she says.

To avoid reinforcing "a system of hierarchical knowledge access," Dr. Headen advises that power dynamics and ownership need to be carefully considered by investigators throughout the research process. "Community-based system dynamics are distinct in that they center the community at the core of any model-building process."

The community-based approach is iterative and designed to empower communities, build capacity, and promote cohesion and long-term engagement. Participants provide input on how they are affected by problems and the interplay among those problems, and then develop models for implementing change in their own environment. The ultimate goal of their involvement, which typically involves multiple projects over time, is to decrease the participatory role of outsiders and foster a sense of local ownership.

"When people are at the table, they're more likely to act on the actual policies or insights or leverage points that are identified from that modeling process," Dr. Headen observes. "The goals are to build shared insight, develop consensus around the factors shaping the problem, and increase motivation for implementing results."

Group Model Building

Community-based system dynamics is a sub-category of group model building, a participatory approach that involves stakeholders in the modeling process. As described by Dr. Headen, group model building advances in several phases[24]:

- **Phase 1: Problem scoping**. Defining the problem is the initial step and requires identifying the main outcome or behavior of interest. This can be done either within the team or by soliciting the ideas and perspectives of leaders across sectors.
- **Phase 2: Core modeling team planning and design**. The second step is to strategically recruit a small set of key stakeholders, including those with lived experience, to form the core modeling team to refine the scope of the problem and design the group model-building sessions. This includes the following tasks:

    - **Script selection**. Pre-developed "scripts" are used to facilitate discussion. These scripts, which can come from sources such as Scriptapedia, are a set of activities across different capacity-building approaches to help a group articulate its understanding of how a system works.[25] The

core modeling team decides how the scripts will be organized to obtain sought-after information and creates a manual to facilitate each session.
   - **Participant recruitment**. Next, the core modeling team, in conjunction with academic researchers, recruits community participants, stakeholders, and facilitators for the group model building workshop and finalizes the structure.

- **Phase 3: Group model-building workshop**. The core modeling team, partnering with facilitators and researchers, implements the scripts during the workshop, which may last over one or several days. The goal is to elicit each participant's "mental models" about the system under discussion (that is, the values, attitudes, and norms that drive their perceptions), as well as the structural factors, relationships, and feedback loops hey perceive to be driving the system's behavior. These can vary based on an individual's position within the system. The goal is to produce a systems map or model that represents the group's consensus on the dynamic mechanisms driving the problem at hand.
- **Phase 4: Model refinement**. In this final phase, the model is refined by the core modeling team and brought back to the group for feedback aligned with the following questions: What did we get right? What did we get wrong? What's here that shouldn't be? What's not here that should be?

Similar to any authentic community-engaged process, the successful use of community-based system dynamics requires relationship-building to develop trust. Researchers need to understand the history of the research that has previously been conducted in a community and the power dynamics associated with it. "Implementing community-based system dynamics is not so different from implementing any type of community-engaged work," says Dr. Headen. "Where it's different is in helping community members learn this new method that visualizes the complexity they know to be at work in the system and then take ownership of it."

Using accessible and experience-based scripts allows community members to see patterns and relationships among the many facets of a problem. When that happens, Dr. Headen says, "You see buy-in because the process is representing the holistic and dynamic perspective that they have, and their experience, in relation to the problem. Once you lay a strong foundation for good community-engaged research practice and step them through a well-facilitated group model-building process, communities get excited about having a system that represents what they know to be true."

The result can be a map illustrating how the community views the connections between different factors, the variables they consider important, and the interwoven relationships as they experience them. Like other types of epidemiological outcomes modeling, it can also generate a simulation model that can be manipulated to see how outcomes are affected.[26] For example, a researcher evaluating the link between an intervention to improve job access and low birthweight can incorporate different options (e.g., adding more jobs, investing in training programs, improving transportation) into a simulation, separately and together, to predict desired impact on inequities.

> These interrelationships may create surprising outcomes when we look at them together rather than separately, —Irene Headen, Drexel Dornsife School of Public Health.

Partners for Advancing Health Equity (P4HE)

Systems science has the potential to take research well beyond the methodological canons Dr. Plough referenced earlier in this chapter. Another strategy to move research in new directions is the research learning collaborative Partners for Advancing Health Equity[27] (P4HE), which brings together researchers, practitioners, community leaders, and policymakers, among others. Through a multi-layered set of activities, events, and resources, the partners learn from one another; share knowledge, skills, and resources; and promote actionable research, practice, and policies. Tulane University School of Public Health and Tropical Medicine leads P4HE, with funding from RWJF.

"The magnitude of the problem that we're addressing is massive," said Dean and P4HE principal investigator Thomas A. LaVeist. "Partnership is a critical part of what is needed to make the changes in society to produce the outcome of health equity that we're interested in." The concept underlying P4HE is to leverage partnerships, bring together resources strategically, and work collaboratively in pursuit of an impact that is larger than would be possible by any individual or sector alone.

P4HE is a membership organization open to anyone committed to "a society where everyone has the ability to live the healthiest life possible." Its activities include:

- **Webinar series.**[28] Different sectors—academia, philanthropy, government, community, and the private sector—often speak different languages even when they are talking about the same ideas. The webinar series is a way to harmonize language and establish a shared level of knowledge and understanding. Examples of recent webinars include "Building Partnerships for Health Equity Advocacy" and "Centering Global & Indigenous Solutions for Health Equity."

- **Workshops**. P4HE workshops consist of three parts: learning about the topic, discussing it, and creating products. Each workshop series addresses a different skills-based topic that supports advancing health equity, offering a place to practice and apply what has been learned. For example, Andrew Anderson, PhD, MPH, from Johns Hopkins University, led a workshop series on defining and measuring success in achieving health equity.
- **Resource library.**[29] Available to anyone through the P4HE website, this library includes tools, reports, and methodologies from a range of organizations and entities engaged with health equity. The library provides researchers, policymakers, and practitioners in real-world settings free access to high-quality research and field-tested, evidence-based programs and strategies.
- **Podcast.**[30] The P4HE podcast provides information on strategies and interventions that have been found to impact health equity. Traditionally, academic research has been disseminated through academic journals that are not easily accessible and generally do not publish negative findings. The P4HE podcast fills a gap by discussing important health equity topics, interventions, challenges, and successes, and also includes conversations with pioneers in health equity research.
- **Convenings**. P4HE brings people together from the many sectors committed to health equity, including academia, community-based organizations, government, philanthropy, and the private sector. The December 2022 "Partners for Advancing Health Equity Summit: On the Front Lines of Equity and Justice,"[31] held in New Orleans, was the first of the planned convenings.

A Final Word

A full understanding of the forces underlying structural racism and its role in health disparities and inequity is key to advancing the goal of offering everyone the opportunity for health and well-being. Data and research methods and models that go beyond conventional strategies can further this understanding.

The contributors to this final chapter offer fresh thinking about how to move beyond the strictures of traditional studies to consider thorny problems in new and more expansive ways. Clear research guidelines emerge from their experiences: approach structural racism head-on, operate across disciplines, make way for the community to lead, think beyond borders of all kinds, embrace new technology in service to equity, use a broad lens to consider what might be relevant, work collaboratively, and be clear on the questions being investigated. All of that should operate in tandem with a willingness to experiment, pivot as new data and information become available, fill a toolbox with multiple tools that fit a range of problems, and bring all parties together to leverage their knowledge, insight, experience, and perspective.

Innovative research models, frameworks, methods, and partnerships can support the actionable knowledge essential to dismantling the pervasive scourge of racism and building health equity. In the current climate, with its many challenges, the enthusiasm and commitment on display offer reason for optimism.

CONCLUSION

Advancing Health for All: On the Front Lines of Equity and Justice opened with the harmony, rhythm, and democratic impulses of jazz, and closed with challenges to the methodological canons of research. Other chapters looked at the environmental perils that menace New Orleans right here, right now, and warned that climate disasters threaten vulnerable populations everywhere. The volume also examined community-driven design and the value of equity commitments in the built environment to curb the damage inflicted by segregation, disinvestment, and exclusionary development. In highlighting racial differences in health outcomes, still another chapter explained how clinical decision-making must be informed by an understanding of race-based oppression, not by mistaken ideas about genetic variability.

The through line in this volume is that RWJF and its partners are reimagining opportunities to generate data and act on the resulting knowledge and thinking in new ways about how best to inspire and sustain transformation. The power imbalances that tilt decision-makers away from equity and justice have led the Foundation to focus ever more on empowering communities to tackle structural racism and other systemic issues. Our animating conviction is that collective action in the most impacted communities enables them to hold decision-makers accountable, drive structural change, and advance health equity.

The historically Black city of New Orleans already has a concentration of committed activists motivated to do just that, and a groundswell of grassroots organizing is evident across the country as well. RWJF has numerous initiatives in place to inform, support, and share their equity-focused efforts. A few examples:

- Partners for Advancing Health Equity Collaborative,[1] launched in 2022 by Tulane University Celia Scott Weatherhead School of Public Health and Tropical Medicine with a $2.9 million RWJF award, is a research learning collaborative that fosters connectivity among scholars, philanthropies, federal research funders, community members, and private sector representatives.

- Since 2017, the Foundation has worked with community leaders in many US cities through its Health and Climate Solutions program[2] to identify and learn from projects that are tackling three intertwined issues—improving health, advancing health equity, and addressing climate change.
- Lead Local Collaborative,[3] which ran from 2018–2020, brought together organizers, advocates, and researchers to consider how local power can catalyze, create, and sustain the conditions needed for healthy communities.

These efforts, and so many others, are built on the belief that cross-cutting partnerships can break down barriers between traditional academic approaches and knowledge embedded in community experience. We think the resulting dialogue is critical to inform new ways of thinking about the drivers of health, the outcomes that get measured, and the action steps necessary to foster equity. With community-developed data in hand, and commitments to collaborate on level ground, we can use science to rebalance knowledge and galvanize the forces of change across community systems and institutions.

ACKNOWLEDGMENTS

Partners for Advancing Health Equity Summit involved the hard work of many talented individuals, both internal and external to the Robert Wood Johnson Foundation. Thank you to Sheldon Watts (RWJF) and Greta Cappelmann (Tulane) for leading the successful development of the summit.

Turning the summit into this volume also required the vision and support of many. An Editorial Review Group oversees the development of this series and provides careful commentary and suggestions. Our colleagues in this group are Sandro Galea, Boston University; Sherry Glied, New York University; Anita Chandra, RAND Corporation; and Sarah Humphreville, Oxford University Press.

Special thanks to the team at RWJF who provided essential leadership and support throughout the development of this manuscript: Ketana Bhavsar, Allyn Brooks-LaSure, and, especially, Kristin Silvani.

Finally, a team of immensely talented writers crafted the manuscript—weaving together multiple narratives, data sources, conference presentations, and extensive interviews into cross-cutting chapters that reflect the themes of the summit. We are so grateful for their rigor, dedication, teamwork, and creativity. Thank you for your exceptional work, Monica L. Coleman, Karyn Feiden, Mary B. Geisz, Margaret O. Kirk, and Mary Nakashian.

Editors:
Alonzo L. Plough, PhD
Thomas A. LaVeist, PhD

NOTES

Prelims

1. Louisiana Department of Health. (2021). *Louisiana health report card.* https://ldh.la.gov/assets/oph/Center-PHI/2021_Health_Report_Card.pdf.
2. Tulane University. (n.d.). *Our patients.* https://medicine.tulane.edu/internal-medicine-residency/our-patients.
3. Chavez R. (2022, July 6). "New Orleans was once the center of U.S. slave trade. This artist wants to make sure we don't forget." *PBS News.* https://www.pbs.org/newshour/arts/new-orleans-was-once-the-center-of-u-s-slave-trade-this-artist-wants-to-make-sure-we-dont-forget.
4. Equal Justice Initiative. (2022). *The Transatlantic Slave Trade.* https://eji.org/report/transatlantic-slave-trade/new-orleans/#a-city-built-on-trafficking.
5. Lewis K. (2020). *A portrait of Louisiana 2020.* https://ssrc-static.s3.amazonaws.com/moa/A_Portrait_of_Louisiana_2020.pdf.
6. https://www.epa.gov/sites/default/files/2019-12/documents/waiting_to_die_final.pdf.

Chapter 1

1. White M. (2010). "Traditional New Orleans jazz as a metaphor for American life." *Imagining America Tenth Annual Conference.* https://imaginingamerica.org/wp-content/uploads/Foreseeable-Futures-9-White.pdf. White M. (2022, December). *New Orleans Jazz as a Metaphor for American Life* [Conference presentation]. Partners for Advancing Health Equity Summit, Tulane University Celia Scott Weatherhead School of Public Health and Tropical Medicine, Tulane, NO, USA.
2. White. "Traditional New Orleans jazz as a metaphor for American life."

Spotlight

1. Fausset R. (2023, February 9). "36 hours in New Orleans," *The New York Times.* https://www.nytimes.com/interactive/2023/02/09/travel/things-to-do-new-orleans.html.
2. Russonello G. (2019, May 28). "After a scandal, the New Orleans Jazz Market rises again." *The New York Times.* https://www.nytimes.com/2019/05/28/arts/music/new-orleans-jazz-market.html.

Chapter 2

1. Elie L. (2019, August 27). "Gentrification might kill New Orleans before climate change does." *The New York Times.*

2. Research and Evaluation Center. (2020). *Reducing violence without police: A review of research evidence*. John Jay College of Criminal Justice, City University of New York.
3. https://healthyneighborhoodsnola.com/.
4. Branas CC, South E, Kondo MC, et al. (2018). "Citywide cluster randomized trial to restore blighted vacant land and its effects on violence, crime, and fear." *Proceedings of the National Academy of Science, 115*(12): 2946–2951.
5. https://www.iwesnola.org/.
6. https://www.evidenceforaction.org/.
7. In sociology, a "third spot" is a place for social interaction separate from the first two spots of home and work. Examples include churches, cafés, libraries, and parks.
8. Task Force on Racial Equity, Diversity, and Inclusion. (2021, February 12). *Final report and recommendations*. Tulane School of Architecture.
9. https://solitarygardens.org/.
10. https://www.sugarrootsfarm.org/.
11. https://parisitediy.com/about-us/.
12. https://maccno.com/guide-to-street-performance-1.
13. https://static1.squarespace.com/static/5839e0cf8419c204f71e961c/t/585c292903596e058c4262c9/1482434859986/MACCNO_street_performance_guide.pdf.
14. Anon. (2019, August 26). "The 1619 Project makes the case . . . Tulane owes African Americans an apology." *The Louisiana Weekly*. http://www.louisianaweekly.com/the-1619-project-makes-the-case-tulane-owes-african-americans-an-apology/.
15. Robinson KK. (2018, May 23). "Walking New Orleans' oldest road." *Curbed New Orleans*.
16. Anon. (2018, January 22). "Bayou Road: The Portage." *WGNO*.
17. http://www.refreshnola.org/.
18. https://www.libertyskitchen.org/.
19. https://goldringcenter.tulane.edu/.
20. https://edibleschoolyard.org/.
21. https://www.sproutnolafarm.org/.
22. https://www.boystown.org/locations/louisiana/Pages/default.aspx.
23. https://www.ccclt.org/.
24. https://www.iseechange.org/.
25. https://floridadep.gov/ResilientFlorida.
26. An example: ISeeChange (2020, August 7). *How ISeeChangers Influenced Stormwater Project Designs in Gentilly*.

Chapter 3

1. The Deep South Center for Environmental Justice. (2021, November 23). *Dr. Beverly Wright talks to Black News Channel about climate change at COP26*. https://www.dscej.org/the-latest/dr-beverly-wright-talks-to-black-news-channel-about-climate-change-at-cop26.
2. National Center for Health Statistics. "Louisiana." October 3, 2024. https://restoredcdc.org/www.cdc.gov/nchs/pressroom/states/louisiana/la.htm
3. The Deep South Center for Environmental Justice. *Surviving Cancer Alley: The stories of five communities*. August 1, 2020. https://fluxconsole.com/files/item/211/109412/SurvivingCancerAlleyReport.pdf.
4. Robert Wood Johnson Foundation. (2022, May 16). *Climate change threatens our health and deepens health inequities*. https://www.rwjf.org/en/insights/our-research/2021/09/climate-change-threatens-our-health-and-deepens-health-inequities.html.
5. United States Environmental Protection Agency. (2021, September 2). *EPA report shows disproportionate impacts of climate change on socially vulnerable populations in the United States*. https://www.epa.gov/newsreleases/epa-report-shows-disproportionate-impacts-climate-change-socially-vulnerable.
6. Woodward, L. (2021, December 16). "How redlining shaped New Orleans' neighborhoods: Is it too late to be fixed?" *Gambit*. https://www.nola.com/

gambit/news/how-redlining-shaped-new-orleans-neighborhoods-is-it-too-late-to-be-fixed/article_215014ce-0c15-5917-b773-8d1d2fdaa655.html.

7. Woodward. "How redlining shaped New Orleans' neighborhoods."
8. Fears D. (2022, April 1). "Gordon Plaza was sold as a dream for Black home buyers. It was a toxic nightmare." *The Washington Post.* https://www.washingtonpost.com/climate-environment/2022/04/01/new-orleans-gordon-plaza-epa/; The Deep-South Center for Environmental Justice. (2022). *Still Growing Strong: 2022 Impact Report.* https://fluxconsole.com/files/item/211/167892/WEB_DSCEJ_FINAL_2023_%20IMPACT_REPORT_V1_3.pdf.
9. Bullard R.D., Wright B. *The wrong complexion for protection.* New York: NYU Press, 2012.
10. Henry J. Kaiser Family Foundation. (2022, May 24). *Climate change and health equity: Key questions and answers.* https://www.kff.org/racial-equity-and-health-policy/issue-brief/climate-change-and-health-equity-key-questions-and-answers/.
11. Robert Wood Johnson Foundation. *Climate Change Threatens our Health and Deepens Health Inequities.*
12. Robert Wood Johnson Foundation. *Climate Change Threatens our Health and Deepens Health Inequities.*
13. A Community Voice ~ Louisiana. *New Orleans' Lower 9th Ward is still reeling from Hurricane Katrina's damage 15 years later.* August 25, 2020. https://www.acommunityvoice.org/category/blight/
14. Henry J. Kaiser Family Foundation. (2007). *Giving voices to the people of New Orleans: The Kaiser post-Katrina baseline survey.* https://www.kff.org/wp-content/uploads/2013/01/7631.pdf.
15. Greater New Orleans Foundation, City of New Orleans, and The DeepSouth Center for Environmental Justice. (2018). *Taking steps together on equity and climate change: A report by and for New Orleanians.* https://issuu.com/greaterneworleansfoundation/docs/2019.08.30_-_climate_action_equity_report_-_web.
16. Robert Wood Johnson Foundation. (2022, November 3). *How unjust policies influence who experiences the harms of climate change first.* https://www.rwjf.org/en/insights/blog/2022/11/how-unjust-policies-influence-who-experiences-the-harms-of-climate-change-first.html.
17. Seaver N., Dryden S., Day-Burget J. (2022). "Barriers and opportunities in communicating about the intersection of health, climate change and equity." *The Journal of Climate Change and Health,* 7. https://doi.org/10.1016/j.joclim.2022.100185.
18. Robert Wood Johnson Foundation. "How unjust policies influence who experiences the harms of climate change first."
19. UNICEF. (2023). *Water scarcity.* https://data.unicef.org.
20. McTeer Toney H. (2023). *Before the streetlights come on: Black America's urgent call for climate solutions.* Minneapolis: Broadleaf Books.
21. Brandes Gratz R. (2013, June 5). "How to save New Orleans from sinking." *The Nation.* https://www.thenation.com/article/archive/how-save-new-orleans-sinking/; Campanella R. (2018, February 6). "How humans sank New Orleans." *The Atlantic.* https://www.theatlantic.com/technology/archive/2018/02/how-humans-sank-new-orleans/552323/. Bittle J. (2023, February 22). "As Louisiana's coast disappears, its historic communities do, too." *Grist.* https://grist.org/migration/louisiana-pointe-aux-chenes-great-displacement-book-excerpt-hurricane-managed-retreat/.
22. RESTORE the Mississippi River Delta. (n.d.). *Sediment diversions.* https://mississippiriverdelta.org/restoration-solutions/sediment-diversions/.
23. Waggonner & Ball. (2013). *Greater New Orleans urban water plan.* https://wbae.com/projects/greater-new-orleans-urban-water-plan-2/.
24. *Gentilly Resilience District: Fact Sheet.* March 1, 2018. Gentilly Resilience District, City of New Orleans. https://nola.gov/archived/resilience-sustainability/resources/fact-sheets/gentilly-factsheet/
25. ByWater Institute. Tulane University. https://bywater.tulane.edu.
26. Campanella. "How humans Sank New Orleans."

27. Smialek J., Swanson A. (2023, January 23). "The death of globalization? You won't find it in New Orleans." *The New York Times*. https://www.nytimes.com/2023/01/20/business/economy/globalization-new-orleans.html.
28. NOAA Fisheries. (2022). *Conducting large-scale wetland restoration in Louisiana*. https://www.fisheries.noaa.gov/national/habitat-conservation/conducting-large-scale-wetland-restoration-louisiana.
29. NOAA Fisheries. *Conducting large-scale wetland restoration in Louisiana*.
30. Schleifstein M. (2021, April 13). "Major Louisiana coastal project encounters new resistance." *Houma Today*. https://www.houmatoday.com/story/news/2021/04/13/major-louisiana-coastal-project-encounters-new-resistance/7210037002/.
31. Louisiana Coastal Protection and Restoration Authority. March 8, 2023. "CPRA Receives NFWF Funding Allocation for Construction of Mid-Barataria Sediment Diversion." https://coastal.la.gov/news/today-the-national-fish-and-wildlife-foundations-nfwf-board-of-directors-approved-the-louisiana-coastal-protection-and-restoration-authoritys-cpra-request-to-dedicate-660-milli/
32. Narayan S., Beck M.W., Wilson P., et al. (2017). "Value of coastal wetlands for flood damage reduction in the Northeastern USA." *Scientific Reports* 7, Article 9463. www.nature.com/articles/s41598-017-09269-z. United States Environmental Protection Agency. (2006). *Wetlands: Protecting life and property from flooding*. www.epa.gov/sites/production/files/2016-02/documents/flooding.pdf.
33. Block W.T. (2000, April 22). "Indians led the way in storm survival." *Beaumont Enterprise*.
34. Smialek and Swanson. "The death of globalization?"
35. National Academies of Sciences, Engineering, Medicine. (2023). *Funding opportunity: Improving public health data systems to address health equity challenges for at-risk communities in the U.S. Gulf Coast*. https://www.nationalacademies.org/our-work/funding-opportunity-improving-public-health-data-systems-to-address-health-equity-challenges-for-at-risk-communities-in-the-us-gulf-coast.
36. The Water Collaborative of Greater New Orleans. "Southeast Louisiana Residential Water Quality Study." Summer 2025. https://drive.google.com/file/d/1nqLxvHR-Nvuz_j-S6kac1fpgXyN5nYsz/view?usp=sharing
37. The DeepSouth Center for Environmental Justice. *Still going strong*.
38. Fausset R. (2023, February 9). "36 hours in New Orleans." *The New York Times*. https://www.nytimes.com/interactive/2023/02/09/travel/things-to-do-new-orleans.html.

Spotlight

1. Robert Wood Johnson Foundation. (n.d.). *Building community power to advance health equity*. https://www.rwjf.org/en/building-a-culture-of-health/focus-areas/Features/building-community-power-to-advance-health-equity.html.

Chapter 4

1. US Department of the Interior: Indian Affairs. *Federal Indian Boarding School Initiative*. May 11, 2022. https://www.bia.gov/service/federal-indian-boarding-school-initiative
2. David J. Sencer CDC Museum (n.d.). *The AIDS epidemic in the United States, 1981-early 1990s*. Centers for Disease Control and Prevention.
3. HIV.gov. *A timeline of HIV and AIDS*. Accessed on December 3, 2025. https://www.hiv.gov/hiv-basics/overview/history/hiv-and-aids-timeline
4. Specter M. (2021, June 7). "How ACT UP changed America." *The New Yorker*. Aizenman N. (2019, February 9). "How to demand a medical breakthrough: Lessons from the AIDS fight." *NPR*. https://www.npr.org/sections/health-shots/2019/02/09/689924838/how-to-demand-a-medical-breakthrough-lessons-from-the-aids-fight.
5. Office of National AIDS Policy. "Announcing the National HIV/AIDS Strategy." July 13, 2010. https://obamawhitehouse.archives.gov/blog/2010/07/13/announcing-national-hivaids-strategy
6. Centers for Disease Control and Prevention. "Ending the HIV Epidemic in the U.S. Goals." Mar. 20, 2024. https://www.cdc.gov/ehe/php/about/goals.html
7. The White House. "Fact Sheet: The Biden-Harris Administration Marks World AIDS Day 2021 With Renewed Commitments to Ending the HIV/AIDS Epidemic by 2030." December

1, 2021. https://bidenwhitehouse.archives.gov/briefing-room/statements-releases/2021/12/01/fact-sheet-the-biden-%E2%81%A0harris-administration-marks-world-aids-day-2021-with-renewed-commitments-to-ending-the-hiv-aids-epidemic-by-2030/

8. https://www.truevolution.org/.
9. Martinez A, Martinez-Beltrán S. (2022, September 8). "A Texas judge rules coverage of anti-HIV medicine violates religious freedom." *NPR.* https://www.npr.org/2022/09/08/1121690478/a-texas-judge-rules-coverage-of-anti-hiv-medicine-violates-religious-freedom.

Chapter 5

1. https://www.lead-local.org/.
2. Robert Wood Johns Foundation. (n.d.). *Lead Local: Exploring community-driven change and the power of collective action.* https://www.rwjf.org/en/grants/grantee-stories/programs/lead-local.html. For additional information from Lead Local, see Farhang L, Morales X. "Building community power to achieve health and racial equity: Principles to guide transformative partnerships with local communities." *NAM Commentary.* Washington, DC: National Academy of Medicine, 2022.
3. Robert Wood Johnson Foundation. (n.d.). *Building community power to advance health equity.* https://www.rwjf.org/en/building-a-culture-of-health/focus-areas/Features/building-community-power-to-advance-health-equity.html.
4. https://www.lead-local.org
5. The Lead Local Collaborative. (2019). *Exploring community-driven change and the power of collective action.* https://www.rwjf.org/content/dam/farm/communication_and_promotion/promotion_or_communication/2020/rwjf462894.
6. Iton A., Ross R., Tamber P.S. (2022). "Building community power to dismantle policy-based structural inequity in population health." *Health Affairs 41*(12). https://www.healthaffairs.org/doi/10.1377/hlthaff.2022.00540.
7. https://austinjustice.org/about/.
8. Jankowski P. (2016, September 4). "Austin police: Teen killed by officer identified as David Joseph, 17." *Austin American-Statesman.* https://www.statesman.com/story/news/2016/09/04/austin-police-teen-killed-by-officer-identified-as-david-joseph-17/10107502007/.
9. Hoffberger C. (2017, December 14). "City council blocks police contract." *The Austin Chronicle.*
10. Hoffberger. "City Council Blocks Police Contract."
11. McMahon S., Moore C. (2019, April 8). "To reform the police, target their union contract." *The New York Times.* https://www.nytimes.com/2019/04/08/opinion/austin-police-union-contract.html
12. Austin American-Statesman. "**City Council approves new Austin police contract." Nov 15, 2018.** https://www.statesman.com/story/news/local/flash-briefing/2018/11/15/city-council-approves-new-austin-police-contract/8358501007/
13. https://www.votersorganized.org/.
14. Sledge M. (2020, December 5). "Jason Williams wins New Orleans DA race, promising new era in prosecutor's office." *New Orleans Times Picayune.* https://www.nola.com/news/courts/jason-williams-wins-new-orleans-da-race-promising-new-era-in-prosecutors-office/article_f044cf7a-368a-11eb-ac4b-0bbdab4e0c09.html.
15. Sledge M. (2021, December 11). "Susan Hutson defeats Marlin Gusman in Orleans parish sheriff's race." *New Orleans Times Picayune/The New Orleans Advocate.* https://www.nola.com/news/politics/susan-hutson-defeats-marlin-gusman-in-orleans-parish-sheriffs-race/article_8d685482-5a0e-11ec-9a37-efa45f6d2c92.html.
16. Cline S. (2022, December 10). "Newcomer wins seat on New Orleans Public Service Commission." *Associated Press.* https://apnews.com/article/2022-midterm-elections-politics-louisiana-baton-rouge-utilities-62ce147befa39e377cd9a48716590d90.
17. https://www.votersorganized.org/book-club.

Chapter 6

1. Villarosa L. (2019, August 14). "Myths about physical racial differences were used to justify slavery—and are still believed by doctors today." *The New York Times Magazine.*

2. Hoffman K.M., Trawalter S., Axt J.R., Norman O.M. (2016). "Racial bias in pain assessment and treatment recommendations, and false beliefs about biological differences between Blacks and Whites." *PNAS, 113*(16): 4296–4430.
3. https://www.genome.gov/human-genome-project.
4. Geronimus A.T. (2023). *Weathering: The Extraordinary Stress of Ordinary Life in an Unjust Society*. New York: Hachette Book Group.
5. Agency for Healthcare Research and Quality. (2018). *National Healthcare Quality & Disparities Report.*
6. Office of Minority Health. (2023). *Diabetes and African Americans.* US Department of Health and Human Services.
7. Office of Minority Health. (2023). *Stroke and African Americans.* US Department of Health and Human Services.
8. Office of Minority Health. (2023). *Heart disease and African Americans.* US Department of Health and Human Services.
9. Office of Minority Health. (2023). *Cancer and African Americans.* US Department of Health and Human Services.
10. Hoyert D.L. (2020). *Maternal mortality rates in the United States, 2020.* National Center for Health Statistics, CDC. For more on the maternal healthcare experience of Black women, see Plough A.L. (2022). "Structural racism in Black maternal healthcare." In *Necessary conversations: Understanding racism as a barrier to achieving health equity.* Princeton, NJ and Oxford: Robert Wood Johnson Foundation and Oxford University Press.
11. Powe N.R. (2021). "The pathogenesis of race and ethnic disparities: Targets for achieving health equity." *Clinical Journal of the American Society of Nephrology, 16*: 806–808.
12. Schwartz R.S. (2001). "Racial profiling in medical research." *The New England Journal of Medicine, 344*: 1392–1393. Phimister E.G. (2003). "Medicine and the racial divide." *The New England Journal of Medicine, 348*: 1081–1082. Cooper R.S., Kaufman J.S., Ward R. (2003). "Race and genomics." *The New England Journal of Medicine, 348*: 1166–1170. Burchard E.G., Ziv E., Coyle N.C. et al. (2003). "The importance of race and ethnic background in biomedical research and clinical practice." *The New England Journal of Medicine, 348*: 1170–1175.
13. Bonham V.L., Sellers S.L., Gallagher T.H. et al. (2009). "Physicians' attitudes toward race, genetics, and clinical medicine." *Genetics in Medicine, 11*(4): 279–286. Frank D.F., Gallagher T.H., Sellers S.L. et al. (2010). "Primary care physicians' attitudes regarding race-based therapies." *Journal of Internal Medicine, 25*(5): 384–389.
14. Cunningham B.A., Bonham V.L., Sellars S.L. et al. (2014). "Physicians' anxiety due to uncertainty and use of race in medical decision-making." *Medical Care, 52*(8): 728–733.
15. Bonham V.L., Sellers S.L., and Woolford S. (2014). "Physicians' knowledge, beliefs, and use of race and human genetic variation: New measures and insights." *BMC Health Services Research, 14*: 456. Bonham V.L., Seller S.L. *Scoring Guide: Race Attributes in Clinical Evaluation (RACE) Scale and Genetic Variation Knowledge Assessment Index (GKAI)*. Apr 29, 2024. https://www.genome.gov/sites/default/files/media/files/2024-04/RACE_and_GKAI_Scoring_Manual_29APR24.pdf
16. Abdallah K.E., Calzone K.A., Jenkins J.F. et al. (2019). "A comparison of physicians' and nurse practitioners' use of race in clinical decision-making." *Ethnicity & Disease, 29*(1): 1–8.
17. Okah E., Cronholm P.F., Crow B. et al. (2023). "Race-based care and beliefs regarding the etiology of racial differences in health outcomes." *American Journal of Preventive Medicine, 64*(4): 477–482.
18. Livingston G., Brown A. (2017, May 18). "Intermarriage in the U.S. 50 years after Loving v. Virginia." *Pew Research Center.*
19. Bryc K., Durand E.Y., Macpherson J.M. et al. (2015). "The genetic ancestry of African Americans, Latinos, and European Americans across the United States." *American Journal of Human Genetics, 96*(1): 37–53.
20. Byeon Y.J.J., Islamaj R., Yeganova L. et al. (2021). "Evolving use of ancestry, ethnicity, and race in genetics research: A survey spanning seven decades." *The American Journal of Human Genetics, 108*: 2215–2223.
21. Christmas J.J., Norris D.M., and Primm A.B. (2024). "Public health and mental health disparities in Black communities." In D.M. Norris and A.B. Primm (Eds.), *Mental health, racism,*

and contemporary challenges of being Black in America (pp. 3–18). Washington: American Psychiatric Association Press.

22. Neighbors H.W., Jackson J., Campbell L., Williams D. (1989). "The influence of racial factors on psychiatric diagnosis: A review and suggestions for research." *Community Mental Health Journal, 25*(4): 301–311.
23. Strakowski S.M., Keck P.E., Arnold L.M. et al. (2003). "Ethnicity and diagnosis in patients with affective disorders." *Journal of Clinical Psychiatry, 64*(7): 747–754.
24. Neighbors H.W., Trierweiler S.J., Ford B.C., Muroff J.R. (2003). "Racial difference in DSM diagnosis using a semi-structured instrument: The importance of clinical judgment in the diagnosis of African Americans." *Journal of Health and Social Behavior, 44*(3): 237–256.
25. Vyas D.A., Eisenstein L.G., Jones D.S. (2020). "Hidden in plain sight: Reconsidering the use of race correction in clinical algorithms." *New England Journal of Medicine, 383*: 874–882.
26. Powe N.R. (2020). "Black kidney function matters: Use or misuse of race?" *Journal of the American Medical Association, 324*(8): 737–738.
27. Powe N.R. (2022). "Race and kidney function: The facts and fix amidst the fuss, fuzziness, and fiction." *Medicine*. 3: 93–97.
28. Jones C.A., McQuillan G.M., Kusek J.W. et al. (1998). "Serum creatinine levels in the US population: Third National Health and Nutrition Examination Survey." *American Journal of Kidney Diseases, 32*(6): 992–999.
29. Powe N.R. (2021). "The pathogenesis of race and ethnic disparities: Targets for achieving health equity." *Clinical Journal of the American Society of Nephrology, 16*: 806–808.
30. Diao J.A., Wu G.J., Taylor H.A. et al. (2021). "Clinical implications of removing race from estimates of kidney function." *JAMA, 325*(2): 184–186.
31. Delgado C., Baweja M., Burrows N.R. et al. (2021). "Reassessing the inclusion of race in diagnosing kidney diseases: An interim report from the NKF-ASN task force." *American Journal of Kidney Diseases, 78*(1): 103–115. Delgado C., Baweja M., Crews, D.C. et al. (2022). "A unifying approach for GFR estimation: Recommendations of the NKF-ASN task force on reassessing the inclusion of race in diagnosing kidney disease." *American Journal of Kidney Diseases, 79*(2): 268–288.
32. Neighbors H.W., Trierweiler S.J., Munday C. et al. (1999). "Psychiatric diagnosis of African Americans: Diagnostic divergence in clinician-structured and semistructured interviewing conditions." *Journal of the National Medical Association, 91*(10): 601–612. Trierweiler S.J., Neighbors H.W., Munday C. et al. (2000). "Clinician attributions associated with the diagnosis of schizophrenia in African American and non-African American patients." *Journal of Consulting & Clinical Psychology*, 68(1): 171–175.
33. National Academies of Sciences, Engineering, and Medicine. 2023. *Using Population Descriptors in Genetics and Genomics Research: A New Framework for an Evolving Field*. Washington, DC: The National Academies Press. https://nap.nationalacademies.org/catalog/26902/using-population-descriptors-in-genetics-and-genomics-research-a-new.

Chapter 7

1. Medicaid.gov. (2025). *June 2025 Medicaid & CHIP enrolment data highlights*. https://www.medicaid.gov/medicaid/program-information/medicaid-and-chip-enrollment-data/report-highlights/index.html.
2. Kaiser Family Foundation. (n.d.). *Births Financed by Medicaid [2023]*. https://www.kff.org/medicaid/state-indicator/births-financed-by-medicaid/?currentTimeframe=0&sortModel=%7B%22colId%22:%22Location%22,%22sort%22:%22asc%22%7D.
3. Congress.gov. (2022, June). *Who Pays for Long-Term Services and Supports?*. https://crsreports.congress.gov/product/pdf/IF/IF10343.
4. Corallo B., Moreno S. (2023, February 6). "Analysis of recent national trends in Medicaid and CHIP enrolment." Kaiser Family Foundation. https://www.kff.org/coronavirus-covid-19/issue-brief/analysis-of-recent-national-trends-in-medicaid-and-chip-enrollment/.
5. Moss K, Dawson S. et al. (2020, March 23). "The Families First Coronavirus Response Act: Summary of key provisions." Kaiser Family Foundation. https://www.kff.org/coronavirus-covid-19/issue-brief/the-families-first-coronavirus-response-act-summary-of-key-provisions/.

6. Somers S., Perkins J. (2022). "The ongoing racial paradox of the Medicaid program." *National Health Law Program.* https://healthlaw.org/resource/the-ongoing-racial-paradox-of-the-medicaid-program/.
7. Somers, Perkins. "The ongoing racial paradox of the Medicaid program."
8. Somers, Perkins. "The ongoing racial paradox of the Medicaid program."
9. Somers, Perkins. "The ongoing racial paradox of the Medicaid program."
10. Office of the Assistant Secretary for Planning and Evaluation. (2023, January 19). *HHS poverty guidelines for 2023.* https://aspe.hhs.gov/topics/poverty-economic-mobility/poverty-guidelines.
11. Kaiser Family Foundation. (2012, August 1). "A guide to the Supreme Court's decision on the ACA's Medicaid expansion." https://www.kff.org/health-reform/issue-brief/a-guide-to-the-supreme-courts-decision/.
12. Medicaid.gov. (n.d.). *Program history and prio initiatives.* https://www.medicaid.gov/about-us/program-history/index.html.
13. Kaiser Family Foundation (2023, March 18). *Status of state Medicaid expansion decisions.* https://www.kff.org/medicaid/issue-brief/status-of-state-medicaid-expansion-decisions-interactive-map/.
14. Somers, Perkins. "The ongoing racial paradox of the medicaid program."
15. CMS Office of Minority Health. (2022, November). *The Path Forward: Improving Data to Advance Health Equity Solutions.* https://www.cms.gov/files/document/path-forwardhe-data-paper.pdf.
16. USA.gov. (n.d.). *Centers for Medicare and Medicaid Services.* https://www.usa.gov/federal-agencies/centers-for-medicare-and-medicaid-services.
17. https://www.cms.gov/files/document/2022-cms-strategic-framework.pdf.
18. https://www.federalregister.gov/documents/2021/01/25/2021-01753/advancing-racial-equity-and-support-for-underserved-communities-through-the-federal-government.
19. https://www.cms.gov/about-cms/agency-information/omh/health-equity-programs/grants-and-awards/health-equity-data-access-program.
20. https://www.cms.gov/about-cms/agency-information/omh/health-equity-programs/rural-health.
21. https://www.cms.gov/about-cms/agency-information/omh/health-equity-programs/grants-and-awards/minority-research-grant-program.
22. https://www.cms.gov/about-cms/agency-information/omh/equity-initiatives/health-equity-technical-assistance.
23. https://www.cms.gov/files/document/cms-framework-health-equity.pdf
24. https://www.cdc.gov/nchs/healthy_people/index.htm.
25. Centers for Medicare & Medicaid Services. "CMS Strategic Framework." Accessed on December 4, 2025. https://www.cms.gov/files/document/cms-strategic-framework-fact-sheet.pdf.
26. US Census Bureau. "LOUISIANA: 2020 Census." August 25, 2021. https://www.census.gov/library/stories/state-by-state/louisiana.html
27. US Census Bureau. (2022, October). *Poverty: 2019 and 2021.* https://www.census.gov/content/dam/Census/library/publications/2022/acs/acsbr22-014.pdf.
28. US Census Bureau (2022, September 13). *Income in the United States 2021.* https://www.census.gov/library/publications/2022/demo/p60-276.html.
29. https://gov.louisiana.gov/assets/ExecutiveOrders/JBE1601.pdf.
30. Louisiana Department of Health. (2022, December). *Medicaid monthly forecast report.* https://ldh.la.gov/assets/medicaid/forecast/2022-Medicaid-Forecast-Report_Dec22.pdf.
31. https://www.kff.org/policy-watch/postpartum-coverage-extension-in-the-american-rescue-plan-act-of-2021/.
32. Louisiana Department of Health. (2021, June 23). *Request for proposals for Louisiana Medicaid managed care organizations.* https://ldh.la.gov/assets/medicaid/RFP_Documents/MCO/RFP2021/RFP/3000017417MCORFP.pdf.
33. Louisiana Department of Health. *Request for proposals,* p. 7.
34. Louisiana Department of Health. *Request for proposals,* p. 31.
35. https://ldh.la.gov/subhome/63.

36. https://ldh.la.gov/assets/cphe/resources/Health-Equity-Roadmap-Phase2.pdf.
37. https://nola.gov/health-department/.
38. City Health Dashboard. "City Overview for New Orleans, LA." Accessed on December 4, 2025. https://www.cityhealthdashboard.com/LA/New%20Orleans/city-overview?tab=demographics_overview
39. Personal correspondence with LA Department of Health, from enrollment records.
40. Tolbert J., Drake P., Damico A. (2022, December 19). *Key facts about the uninsured population.* San Francisco: Kaiser Family Foundation. https://www.kff.org/uninsured/issue-brief/key-facts-about-the-uninsured-population/.

Spotlight

1. Medicaid and CHIP Payment and Access Commission. "Availability of Race and Ethnicity Data for Medicaid Beneficiaries." March 2022. https://www.macpac.gov/wp-content/uploads/2022/03/MACPAC-brief_Race-and-Ethnicity-Data-Availability.pdf
2. CMS Office of Minority Health. *The Path Forward.*
3. Louisiana Department of Health. *Request for proposals.*

Chapter 8

1. https://www.rwjf.org/en/insights/our-research/2021/10/charting-a-course-for-an-equity-centered-data-system.html
2. Christopher G.C., Zimmerman E.B., Chandra A., Martin L.T. (2021, October 1). *Charting a Course for an Equity-Centered Data System.* Princeton, NJ: Robert Wood Johnson Foundation.
3. https://www.cdc.gov/places/index.html.
4. https://www.nationalacademies.org/our-work/funding-opportunity-improving-public-health-data-systems-to-address-health-equity-challenges-for-at-risk-communities-in-the-us-gulf-coast.
5. https://debeaumont.org/made-for-health-justice/.
6. https://www.rwjf.org/en/grants/active-funding-opportunities/2023/health-equity-scholars-for-action.html.
7. https://healthpolicyresearch-scholars.org/.
8. https://www.rwjf.org/en/insights/our-research/2022/05/necessary-conversations--we-need-to-talk-about-race-health-and-equity.html
9. https://healourcommunities.org/?gclid=Cj0KCQjw4NujBhC5ARIsAF4Iv6fJaEvxIVAPuAGCwMuPGKwDT5EF3Bhhqf_6wIa4lyx3qjTG2CZVnGYaAuEsEALw_wcB
10. https://healourcommunities.org/
11. Brownell M.D., Chartier M.J., Nickel N.C. et al. (2016). "Unconditional prenatal income supplement and birth outcomes." *Pediatrics, 137*(6). https://publications.aap.org/pediatrics/article-abstract/137/6/e20152992/52383/Unconditional-Prenatal-Income-Supplement-and-Birth?redirectedFrom=fulltext
12. Hardy B.L., Collyer S.M., Wimer C. (2023, March). *The Antipoverty Effects of the Expanded Child Tax Credit across States: Where Were the Historic Reductions Felt?* Washington, CD: The Brookings Institution.
13. https://www.hopeinitiative.org/about.
14. The HOPE Initiative is led by the National Collaborative for Health Equity and Texas Health Institute in partnership with Virginia Commonwealth University's Center on Society and Health and is funded by the Robert Wood Johnson Foundation.
15. Diez Roux A.V. (2011). "Complex systems thinking and current impasses in health disparities research." *American Journal of Public Health, 101*: 1627–1634. Sterman JD. (2006). "Learning from evidence in a complex world." *American Journal of Public Health, 96*: 505–514.
16. Meadows D.H. (2008). *Thinking in systems: A primer.* White River Junction, VT: Chelsea Green Publishing.
17. Frerichs L., Hasmiller Lich K., Dave G., Corbie-Smith G. (2016). "Integrating systems science and community-based participatory research to achieve health equity." *American Journal of Public Health, 106*: 215–222. Calancie L., Batdorf-Barnes A., Verbiest S. et al. (2022).

"Practical approaches for promoting health equity in communities." *Maternal and Child Health Journal, 26*(Suppl 1): 82–87.

18. Bonett S., Meanley S., Stevens R. et al. (2020). "The role of networks in racial disparities in HIV incidence among men who have sex with men in the United States." *AIDS and Behavior, 24*(10): 2781–2796.
19. Stojanovski K., King E.J., Amico K.R. et al. (2022). "Stigmatizing policies interact with mental health and sexual behaviours to structurally induce HIV diagnoses among European men who have sex with men." *AIDS and Behavior, 26*(10): 3400–3410.
20. https://www.covidence.org/.
21. https://kumu.io/.
22. Millett G.A., Peterson J.L., Flores S.A. et al. (2012). "Comparisons of disparities and risks of HIV infection in Black and other men who have sex with men in Canada, UK, and USA: A meta-analysis." *Lancet, 380*(9839): 341–348.
23. Goedel W.C., King M.R.F., Lurie M.N. et al. (2018). "Effect of racial inequities in pre-exposure prophylaxis use on racial disparities in HIV incidence among men who have sex with men: A modeling study." *Journal of Acquired Immune Deficiency Syndrome, 79*(3): 323–329.
24. Hovmand P. (2014). *Community-based system dynamics*. New York: Springer-Verlag. Andersen D.F., Richardson G.P. (1997). "Scripts for group model building." *System Dynamics Review, 13*(2):108–129.
25. Scriptapedia is an open access Wiki book that provides comprehensive background information and examples to support this work. See: Hovmand P.S., Rouwette E.A.J.A., Andersen D., Richardson G.P. et al. (n.d.) *Scriptapedia: A handbook of scripts for developing structured group model building sessions,* https://en.wikibooks.org/wiki/Scriptapedia; and Hovmand P.S., Rouwette E.A.J.A. (2014, July). *Scriptapedia 5.0: A tool for designing "scripted" group model building workshops.*
26. Jackson J.W., Arah O.A. (2020). "Invited commentary: Making causal inference more social and (social) epidemiology more causal." *American Journal of Epidemiology, 189*(3): 179–182. Blakely T., Lynch J., Simons K. et al. (2020). "Reflection on modern methods: When worlds collide—prediction, machine learning and causal inference." *International Journal of Epidemiology, 49*(6): 2058–2064.
27. https://www.partners4healthequity.org/.
28. https://www.partners4healthequity.org/resource-library?search=p4he&sort_bef_combine=search_api_relevance_DESC&f%5B0%5D=reference_type%3AWebinar.
29. https://www.partners4healthequity.org/resource-library.
30. https://www.partners4healthequity.org/resource-library?search=p4he&sort_bef_combine=search_api_relevance_DESC&f%5B0%5D=reference_type%3APodcast.
31. https://sph.tulane.edu/partners-health-equity-summit.

Conclusion

1. https://www.partners4healthequity.org/.
2. https://www.rwjf.org/en/insights/our-research/2020/06/the-intersection-of-health-equity-and-climate-change.html
3. https://www.lead-local.org/.

INDEX

For the benefit of digital users, indexed terms that span two pages (e.g., 52–53) may, on occasion, appear on only one of those pages.